Handbook for Venous Thromboembolism

Gregory Piazza • Benjamin Hohlfelder
Samuel Z. Goldhaber

Handbook for Venous Thromboembolism

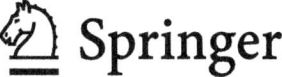 Springer

Gregory Piazza
Cardiovascular Division
Harvard Medical School
Brigham and Women's Hospital
Boston, Massachusetts
USA

Samuel Z. Goldhaber
Thrombosis Research Group
Harvard Medical School
Brigham and Women's Hospital
Boston, Massachusetts
USA

Benjamin Hohlfelder
Department of Pharmacy Services
Brigham and Women's Hospital
Boston, Massachusetts
USA

ISBN 978-3-319-20842-8   ISBN 978-3-319-20843-5   (eBook)
DOI 10.1007/978-3-319-20843-5

Library of Congress Control Number: 2015948376

Springer Cham Heidelberg New York Dordrecht London
© Springer International Publishing Switzerland 2015

Printed on acid-free paper

Springer International Publishing AG Switzerland is part of Springer Science+Business Media
(www.springer.com)

The authors dedicate this book to their mentors, colleagues, and families for their inspiration, guidance, and support.

Preface

Venous thromboembolism (VTE), including deep vein thrombosis (DVT) and pulmonary embolism (PE), is the third most common cardiovascular disorder after myocardial infarction (MI) and stroke. Unlike MI and stroke, which occur most commonly in older patients with numerous medical comorbid conditions, VTE afflicts both the young and old and the seemingly healthy and chronically infirmed. Diagnosis and management of VTE cross the boundaries of many disciplines of medicine. PE and DVT are common complications of major surgery, trauma, cancer, and hospitalization for medical illness. VTE is also an important women's health concern, especially during and after pregnancy and with use of hormonal contraceptive or replacement therapy. Accordingly, an understanding of the risk factors, pathophysiology, diagnosis, treatment, and prevention of VTE is critical for most clinicians, not only cardiovascular medicine specialists.

Over the past three decades, the Brigham and Women's Hospital (BWH) Thrombosis Research Group has focused on advancing patient care and clinical investigation in the field of VTE. From epidemiological studies that have promoted our greater understanding of risk factors to pivotal trials of fibrinolytic therapy for treatment of acute PE and computerized decision support to prevent VTE in high-risk patients, the BWH Thrombosis Research Group has sought to bring the breakthroughs in clinical research to the bedside. More than a decade ago, we were approached by our Healthcare System leadership and asked to draft a set of evidence-based clinical practice guidelines that would help our clinicians navigate the rapid advances in VTE diagnosis, management, and prevention. In response, we drafted the first edition of the *Venous Thromboembolism Guidebook*.

Because the field of VTE has evolved, we have published online and in print five subsequent editions of the *Venous Thromboembolism Guidebook*. The emergence of the non-vitamin K oral anticoagulants and new catheter-based techniques for treatment of DVT and PE have presented an ongoing challenge to clinicians at our medical center, throughout the USA, and worldwide. We are delighted to bring our decades of experience and expertise in evaluation and treatment of patients with VTE to a wider audience in the form of this *Handbook of Venous Thromboembolism*.

In the Handbook, we provide a state-of-the-art but practical guide to understanding the risk factors and pathophysiology, diagnosis and risk stratification, and treatment and prevention of VTE. We use clinical vignettes and self-assessment questions to emphasize key concepts from each chapter. We hope that this *Handbook of Venous Thromboembolism* will enable readers to incorporate changes in our rapidly advancing field into the daily care of patients who have suffered or are at risk for developing VTE.

Boston, MA, USA   Gregory Piazza, MD, MS

Contents

Abbreviations

aPTT	Activated partial thromboplastin time
CT	Computed tomogram
DVT	Deep vein thrombosis
INR	International normalized ratio
IV	Intravenous
IVC	Inferior vena cava
LMWH	Low molecular weight heparin
LV	Left ventricle
MR	Magnetic resonance
NOAC	Non-vitamin K oral anticoagulant
PCC	Prothrombin-complex concentrate
PE	Pulmonary embolism
PTS	Post-thrombotic syndrome
RV	Right ventricle
SC	Subcutaneous
VTE	Venous thromboembolism

Chapter 1
Overview and Epidemiology of Venous Thromboembolism

Abstract Venous Thromboembolism (VTE), including deep vein thrombosis (DVT) and pulmonary embolism (PE), is the third most common cardiovascular disorder after myocardial infarction and stroke. VTE is a common complication of hospitalization and is the most preventable cause of death among hospitalized patients. While the majority of patients who develop VTE do so as outpatients, many have been hospitalized for medical or surgical illness within 3 months preceding the diagnosis of VTE. VTE is frequently a recurrent disease, with patients who suffer unprovoked VTE having the highest risk of future events.

Keywords Deep vein thrombosis • Incidence • Mortality • Pulmonary embolism • Venous thromboembolism

Self-Assessment Questions

1. A 62-year-old woman with a past medical history of hypertension and hyperlipidemia presented with acute right-sided calf pain and ankle edema. She denied any recent major trauma, major surgery, or immobility. A lower extremity venous ultrasound was performed to evaluate for deep vein thrombosis (DVT) and confirmed thrombosis of the right popliteal vein. She has no prior history of venous thromboembolism and is up-to-date with all of her age appropriate cancer screening. Which of the following statements about her risk of VTE recurrence is correct?

    (a) She has a 20 % risk of VTE recurrence over the next 10 years after completing 6 months of anticoagulation for her unprovoked DVT.
    (b) She has a 20 % risk of VTE recurrence over the next 10 years if she remains on indefinite duration anticoagulation after her unprovoked DVT.
    (c) She has a 30–50 % risk of VTE recurrence over the next 10 years after completing 6 months of anticoagulation for her unprovoked DVT.
    (d) She has a 30–50 % risk of VTE recurrence over the next 10 years if she remains on indefinite duration anticoagulation after her unprovoked DVT.

© Springer International Publishing Switzerland 2015
G. Piazza et al., *Handbook for Venous Thromboembolism*,
DOI 10.1007/978-3-319-20843-5_1

2. Which of the following statements about the epidemiology of venous thrombo-embolism (VTE) is false?

   (a) Pulmonary embolism (PE) is the most preventable cause of death among hospitalized medical patients.
   (b) VTE is the third most common cardiovascular disorder after myocardial infarction and stroke.
   (c) Long-term mortality in patients who have suffered an initial VTE is similar to that of age-matched individuals from the general population.
   (d) Recurrent PE is an important cause of mortality in patients who have suf-fered an initial VTE.

Clinical Vignette

A 72-year-old man with prior history of right lower extremity deep vein thrombosis (DVT) following right knee arthroscopy 10 years prior developed acute pleuritic pain and dyspnea at rest while hospitalized for an exacerbation of chronic obstructive pulmonary disease. He had been prescribed venous thromboembolism (VTE) prophylaxis in the form of enoxaparin 40 mg sub-cutaneously daily but had been refusing the injections. Physical examination was remarkable for a resting tachycardia of 108 beats per minute, normal blood pressure of 128/62 mmHg, and hypoxemia with an oxygen saturation on room air of 88 %. He had mild left lower extremity edema. A contrast-enhanced chest computed tomogram (CT) demonstrated bilateral pulmonary embolism (PE) (Fig. 1.1). Lower extremity venous ultrasound demonstrated left common femoral DVT (Fig. 1.2).

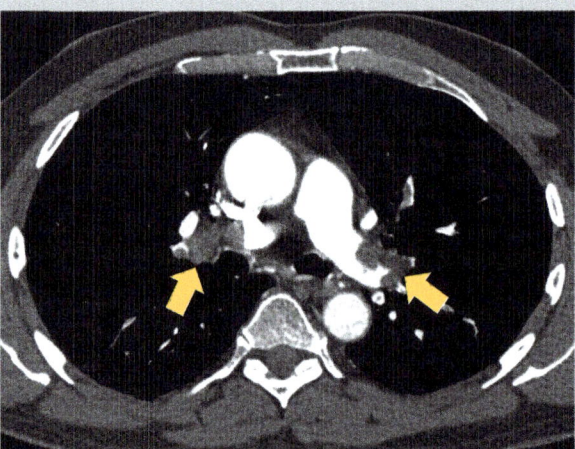

Fig. 1.1 Contrast-enhanced chest computed tomogram (CT) demonstrating bilateral pul-monary embolism (PE) (*arrows*) in a 72-year-old man who developed acute pleuritic pain and dyspnea at rest during a hospitalization for chronic obstructive pulmonary disease

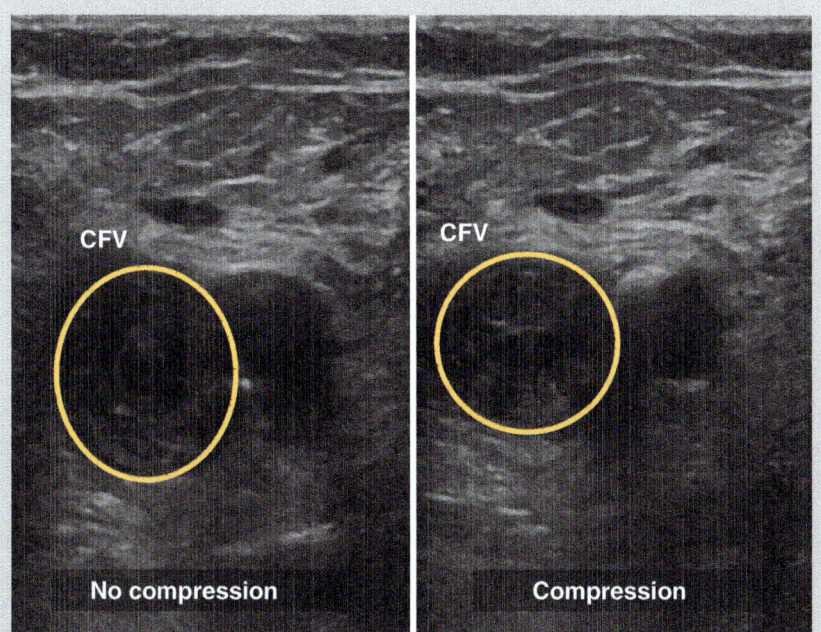

Fig. 1.2 Venous ultrasound demonstrating non-compressibility of the left common femoral vein (*CFV*) consistent with the diagnosis of acute deep vein thrombosis (DVT) in a 72-year-old man who developed acute pulmonary embolism (PE) during an admission for chronic obstructive pulmonary disease. Echogenic material in the lumen of the CFV (*ovals*) represents the presence of thrombus

Venous thromboembolism (VTE), including deep vein thrombosis (DVT) and pulmonary embolism (PE), comprises the third most common cardiovascular disorder after myocardial infarction and stroke [1, 2]. The incidence of VTE rises sharply after age 60 for both men and women, and PE accounts for the majority of this increase [3]. In a population-based analysis of 5025 Worcester, Massachusetts metropolitan area residents, age- and sex-adjusted annual event rates for first-time VTE increased from 73 per 100,000 in 1985 and 1986 to 133 per 100,000 in 2009, primarily due to an increase in PE [4]. In another comparative epidemiological analysis of data from 1998 to 2005, the number of patients with primary or secondary PE on discharge from the hospital increased from 126,546 to 229,637, while the hospital case fatality rate decreased from 12.3 to 8.2 % [5]. Increased sensitivity of diagnostic imaging and enhanced detection of small pulmonary emboli with relatively more benign prognosis may explain, at least in part, the rising incidence and declining mortality of PE. An increase in the number of patients with permanent pacemaker and internal cardiac defibrillator leads, as well as chronic indwelling central venous catheters, has led to a rise in the frequency of upper extremity DVT. The growing epidemic of obesity is another important contributor to the increasing incidence of VTE.

VTE is a common complication of hospitalization for medical and surgical illness. United States Surgeon General's Call To Action To Prevent DVT and PE estimated that 100,000–180,000 deaths occur annually from PE in the U.S. alone and identified PE as the most preventable cause of death among hospitalized patients [6]. While the majority of patients who develop VTE do so as outpatients, many have been hospitalized for medical or surgical illness within 3 months preceding the diagnosis of VTE [7].

The age- and sex-adjusted annual rate of recurrent venous thromboembolism decreased from 39 (95 % confidence interal [CI], 32–45) in 1985 and 1986 to 19 (95 % CI, 15–23) in 2003, and then increased to 35 (95 % CI, 29–40) in 2009 [4]. Patients with unprovoked (idiopathic) VTE have an increased risk of recurrent events following completion of anticoagulation compared with those who have identifiable provoking factors [8, 9]. While the rate of VTE recurrence ranges 30–50 % over 10 years for unprovoked VTE, recurrent events may occur in as many as 20 % of patients over 10 years after a provoked event [8, 9]. The Clinical Vignette above illustrates the recurrent nature of VTE even in those with provoked initial events.

Despite advances in the care of patients with VTE, the in-hospital mortality of patients with acute PE is estimated to be nearly 7 % overall and as high as 32 % for those with hemodynamic instability [10]. An analysis of the Danish National Registry of Patients demonstrated that patients who have suffered an initial episode of VTE have an increased mortality over 30 years of follow-up [11]. Recurrent PE remained an important cause of death throughout this period of increased mortality.

Answer Key

1. **Correct answer**, (**c**) The patient has suffered an unprovoked (idiopathic) DVT. Epidemiological studies have consistently demonstrated a 30–50 % risk of VTE recurrence after an initial event after completion of standard duration anticoagulation (6 months).
2. **Correct answer**, (**c**) A population-wide epidemiological study demonstrated that long-term mortality remains increased for at least 30 years following an initial VTE compared with individuals who have not suffered VTE.

References

1. Glynn RJ, Danielson E, Fonseca FA, et al. A randomized trial of rosuvastatin in the prevention of venous thromboembolism. N Engl J Med. 2009;360:1851–61.
2. Ridker PM, Danielson E, Fonseca FA, et al. Rosuvastatin to prevent vascular events in men and women with elevated C-reactive protein. N Engl J Med. 2008;359:2195–207.
3. Silverstein MD, Heit JA, Mohr DN, Petterson TM, O'Fallon WM, Melton LJ. Trends in the incidence of deep vein thrombosis and pulmonary embolism: a 25-year population-based study. Arch Intern Med. 1998;158:585–93.

4. Huang W, Goldberg RJ, Anderson FA, Kiefe CI, Spencer FA. Secular trends in occurrence of acute venous thromboembolism: the Worcester VTE study (1985–2009). Am J Med. 2014;127:829–39.
5. Park B, Messina L, Dargon P, Huang W, Ciocca R, Anderson FA. Recent trends in clinical outcomes and resource utilization for pulmonary embolism in the United States: findings from the nationwide inpatient sample. Chest. 2009;136:983–90.
6. The surgeon general's call to action to prevent deep vein thrombosis and pulmonary embolism. U.S. Department of Health and Human Services. 2008. Available at: www.ncbi.nlm.nih.gov/books/NBK44178/. Accessed 21 Sept 2014.
7. Spencer FA, Lessard D, Emery C, Reed G, Goldberg RJ. Venous thromboembolism in the outpatient setting. Arch Intern Med. 2007;167:1471–5.
8. Martinez C, Cohen AT, Bamber L, Rietbrock S. Epidemiology of first and recurrent venous thromboembolism: a population-based cohort study in patients without active cancer. Thromb Haemost. 2014;112:255–63.
9. Prandoni P, Noventa F, Ghirarduzzi A, et al. The risk of recurrent venous thromboembolism after discontinuing anticoagulation in patients with acute proximal deep vein thrombosis or pulmonary embolism. A prospective cohort study in 1,626 patients. Haematologica. 2007;92:199–205.
10. Casazza F, Becattini C, Bongarzoni A, et al. Clinical features and short term outcomes of patients with acute pulmonary embolism. The Italian Pulmonary Embolism Registry (IPER). Thromb Res. 2012;130:847–52.
11. Sogaard KK, Schmidt M, Pedersen L, Horvath-Puho E, Sorensen HT. 30-year mortality after venous thromboembolism: a population-based cohort study. Circulation. 2014;130:829–36.

Chapter 2
Risk Factors for Venous Thromboembolism: Recognizing the Spectrum of Risk and Understanding the Role of Thrombophilia Testing

Abstract Risk factors for venous thromboembolism (VTE) include inherited thrombophilias, lifestyle-related risk factors, and acquired conditions of endothelial injury, stasis, and hypercoagulability. The majority of VTE patients presents with a combination of multiple risk factors that result in venous thrombosis. Common acquired risk factors include advanced age, malignancy, immobility, inflammation, and recent trauma, surgery, and hospitalization. Thrombophilia testing is most helpful when the results will assist in decision-making for prevention or treatment of VTE.

Keywords Hypercoagulable states • Risk factors • Thrombophilia • Venous thromboembolism

Self-Assessment Questions

1. Which of the following factors increases the risk of recurrent venous thromboembolism (VTE)?

    (a) Factor V Leiden heterozygosity
    (b) Prothrombin gene mutation homozygosity
    (c) Compound heterozygosity for Factor V Leiden and prothrombin gene mutation
    (d) Suffering an idiopathic (unprovoked) VTE

2. Thrombophilia testing is indicated in which of the following clinical scenarios?

    (a) A 82-year-old man with pulmonary embolism (PE) after a fall complicated by a right hip fracture
    (b) A 56-year-old woman with left lower extremity deep vein thrombosis (DVT) following right mastectomy for breast cancer
    (c) The younger sister of a 23-year-old non-smoking woman with left calf DVT following initiation of a combination oral contraceptive pill
    (d) A 19-year-old collegiate baseball pitcher with right upper extremity DVT following spring training sessions

© Springer International Publishing Switzerland 2015
G. Piazza et al., *Handbook for Venous Thromboembolism*,
DOI 10.1007/978-3-319-20843-5_2

3. Which of the following problems with thrombophilia testing may occur during the acute diagnosis and treatment phase of a patient with PE?

   (a) A false positive result for prothrombin gene mutation testing
   (b) A false negative result for factor V Leiden mutation testing
   (c) A false positive result for protein S deficiency
   (d) A false negative result for protein C deficiency

Clinical Vignette

A 68-year-old woman with past medical history of hypertension and coronary artery disease status post coronary artery bypass graft surgery 5 years prior developed left leg discomfort and edema 1 week following discharge from the hospital for community acquired pneumonia. She was obese and an active smoker. She admitted to spending most of her time in bed watching television since returning home from the hospital. In the Emergency Department, a venous ultrasound demonstrated left popliteal vein DVT (Fig. 2.1).

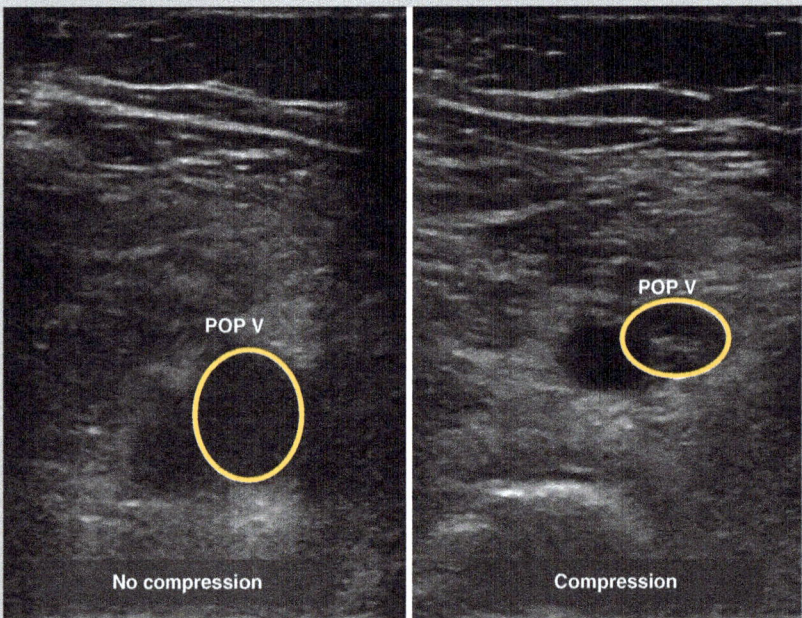

Fig. 2.1 Venous ultrasound demonstrating non-compressibility of the left popliteal vein (*POP V*) (*ovals*) consistent with the diagnosis of acute deep vein thrombosis (DVT) in a 68-year-old woman recently discharged from the hospital after admission for pneumonia who had risk factors for venous thromboembolism (VTE) including obesity, smoking, immobility, coronary artery disease, and age

Recognition of risk factors is a critical step in the assessment of a patient's risk for developing an initial VTE and recurrent events. Inherited thrombophilias, lifestyle-related risk factors, and acquired conditions of endothelial injury, stasis, and hypercoagulability contribute to an individual's risk for VTE (Table 2.1). The majority of patients with VTE presents with a combination of multiple risk factors that result in venous thrombosis. Illustrating this point, the patient in the Clinical Vignette has numerous VTE risk factors, including hypertension, coronary artery disease, obesity, smoking, immobility, and recent acute infectious illness.

Table 2.1 Major risk factors for venous thromboembolism (VTE)

Inherited
Factor V Leiden mutation (activated protein C resistance)
Prothrombin gene mutation 20210
Deficiency of protein C, protein S, or antithrombin
Family history of VTE
Lifestyle
Smoking
Obesity
Diet (high red meat, low fish and vegetable consumption)
Stress
Acquired
Advancing age
Prior history of VTE
Recent surgery, trauma, or hospitalization
Long-haul air travel
Malignancy
Hyperhomocysteinemia (less commonly inherited secondary to a mutation in methylenetetrahydrofolate reductase)
Pregnancy, oral contraceptive pills, or hormone replacement therapy
Atherosclerotic cardiovascular disease and associated factors (including diabetes, dyslipidemia, hypertension)
Pacemaker or implantable cardiac defibrillator leads and indwelling venous catheters
Chronic medical illness (including heart failure, chronic obstructive pulmonary disease, chronic kidney disease)
Lupus anticoagulant, antiphospholipid antibodies, anti-β_2 glycoprotein-1 antibodies, or anticardiolipin antibodies
Immobility
Inflammatory
Acute infectious illness
Blood transfusion and erythropoiesis-stimulating agents
Chronic inflammation (including systemic vasculitides, inflammatory bowel disease)

Inherited Thrombophilias

Inherited thrombophilias should be suspected in patients with VTE at a young age, multiple family members with VTE, VTE in unusual locations, idiopathic or recurrent VTE, or a history of recurrent miscarriages. The prevalence of specific inherited thrombophilias varies according to population demographics. In the general population, inherited thrombophilias are less frequent than "traditional" VTE risk factors, such as cancer, immobility, and obesity [1]. However, in patients who have experienced an initial episode of VTE or have a family history of VTE, the prevalence of inherited thrombophilia increases.

Testing for inherited thrombophilias is often performed to assess the risk of recurrent VTE in a patient with an initial event. However, only a subset of inherited thrombophilias significantly increase the risk of VTE recurrence. While deficiencies of protein C, protein S, or antithrombin consistently increase the risk of recurrent VTE, more common inherited thrombophilias such as factor V Leiden and the prothrombin gene mutation do not appear to increase the risk of recurrence [2]. In a study evaluating the impact of factor V Leiden and the prothrombin gene mutation on VTE recurrence, heterozygosity for either factor V Leiden or the prothrombin gene mutation was not associated with an increased risk of VTE recurrence [3]. Furthermore, compound heterozygosity and homozygosity for either factor V Leiden or prothrombin gene mutation did not increase the risk of recurrent VTE.

Lifestyle-Related Risk Factors

Smoking is a particularly potent VTE risk factor, doubling the risk of unprovoked PE for women who smoke 25–34 cigarettes daily and tripling the risk for those who smoke 35 or more cigarettes daily compared with never-smokers [4]. In a meta-analysis of 63,552 patients from 21 studies, obesity was associated with a doubling in VTE risk [5]. Diets that limit red meat consumption and are rich in fish and vegetables are associated with a lower risk of VTE [6]. Persistently high stress levels are associated with an increased risk of PE [7].

Acquired Risk Factors

Advanced age, malignancy, immobility, and recent trauma, surgery, and hospitalization are well-recognized acquired VTE risk factors. Antiphospholipid antibodies, including the lupus anticoagulant, anticardiolipin antibodies, anti-prothombin antibodies, and anti-β_2 glycoprotein-1 antibodies, are potent acquired risk factors for both venous and arterial thromboembolism. Pregnancy, hormonal contraceptive techniques, and hormone replacement therapy are important VTE risk factors in women. Atherosclerosis and VTE share common pathophysiological processes of inflammation, hypercoagulability, and endothelial injury [8, 9]. Accordingly, atherosclerotic cardiovascular disease and its risk factors are now recognized as important risk factors for VTE [5, 9].

The role of inflammation as a risk factor for VTE has long been suspected on the basis of the observation of an increased frequency of DVT and PE in patients with chronic inflammatory disorders such as systemic vasculitis and inflammatory bowel disease. Acute infectious illness, blood transfusion, and erythropoiesis-stimulating agents have been associated with an increased risk of hospitalization for VTE [10]. The postulated mechanism is systemic inflammation which triggers thrombosis [11]. Elevations in C-reactive protein (CRP), a sensitive marker of systemic inflammation, have been linked to an increased risk of VTE [12]. Polymorphisms in genes encoding factor VII, interleukin-1β, and interleukin-10 modulate the risk of idiopathic VTE [13]. The presence of platelets, neutrophils, and neutrophil extracellular traps (NETs) in human venous thrombus further highlights the importance of inflammation to the development of VTE [14]. In an analysis of the randomized controlled Justification for the Use of Statins in Prevention: an Intervention Trial Evaluating Rosuvastatin (JUPITER) study, rosuvastatin 20 mg orally daily reduced the rate of new onset symptomatic VTE by 43 % in an initially healthy population without hyperlipidemia but with evidence of chronic systemic inflammation as defined by an elevated CRP [15].

Chronic medical conditions, such as heart failure [16, 17] and chronic obstructive pulmonary disease [18], also contribute to the risk of VTE.

Thrombophilia Evaluation

Testing for hypercoagulable states is most useful when the results will assist in decision-making for prevention or treatment of VTE. Thrombophilia testing is often considered in patients with VTE at a young age, recurrent VTE, thrombosis in unusual sites, those with venous and arterial thromboembolism, strong family history of VTE, and recurrent pregnancy loss. The rationale for performing thrombophilia evaluations includes selecting the optimal agent and duration of anticoagulation, predicting the risk of VTE recurrence, determining the optimal intensity of thromboprophylaxis, assessing VTE risk with pregnancy or hormonal contraceptive or replacement therapy, and identifying family members at risk for thrombosis. Patients seeking an explanation for an arterial or venous thrombosis, especially if unprovoked or unexpected, will often request thrombophilia testing. The patient in the Clinical Vignette has multiple risk factors to explain her episode of VTE and would not require a thrombophilia work-up on clinical grounds.

A stepwise strategy for thrombophilia testing that considers the clinical scenario (when to test), the implications of testing (why to test), and then the overall approach

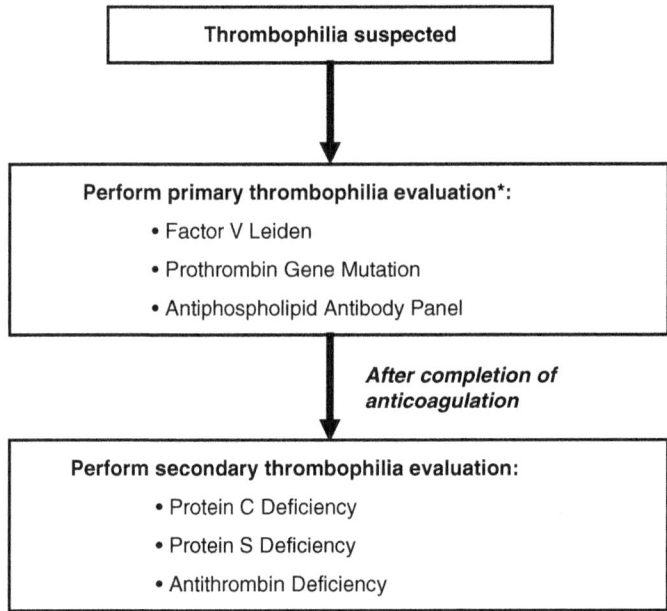

*Can be drawn in the setting of acute thromboembolism or anticoagulation

Fig. 2.2 A stepwise approach to thrombophilia testing

to testing (how to test) is often the most useful (Fig. 2.2). A selective strategy begins with an initial thrombophilia evaluation focused on the highest yield testing, factor V Leiden mutation, prothrombin gene mutation, and antiphospholipid antibodies. Although antiphospholipid antibodies require confirmation 12 weeks after an initial positive result, polymorphisms detected on genetic testing for factor V Leiden or prothrombin gene mutation represent true positives, regardless of when the testing is performed. A secondary evaluation for less common thrombophilias, such as deficiencies of protein C, protein S, and antithrombin, may be performed after completion of anticoagulation if a high index of suspicion for thrombophilia exists and the initial laboratory panel is negative. Because low levels of protein C, protein S, and antithrombin may be observed in the setting of acute thrombosis and anticoagulation and do not necessarily indicate true thrombophilia, testing for these thrombophilias should be deferred acutely (Table 2.2).

   Although the desire to perform thrombophilia testing during the patient's acute hospitalization for VTE is frequently high, a strong case can be made to defer evaluation to the follow-up outpatient visit. Clinicians often have limited time and resources during the hectic hospitalization for VTE to explain the implications of a thrombophilia diagnosis on management and to answer related questions. In addition, the psychological shock of suffering thrombosis may hinder a patient's ability to absorb the implications of a discussion regarding thrombophilia testing and its ramifications.

Table 2.2 Clinical pearls for thrombophilia testing

Follow a stepwise approach for thrombophilia testing that considers the clinical scenario (when to test), the implications of testing (why to test), and a selective strategy for testing (how to test)
A selective strategy emphasizes the highest yield thrombophilia testing first given the individual patient's demographics and presentation
Defer testing for deficiencies of protein C, protein S, and antithrombin because low levels do not necessarily indicate true thrombophilia in the setting of acute thromboembolism and in the presence of anticoagulant therapy
Remind patients that a negative thrombophilia evaluation does not exclude thrombophilia since there are many hypercoagulable conditions that have yet to be identified and for which routine testing does not exist
Defer thrombophilia testing to the follow-up outpatient visit when there will be more time available for interactive discussion and patient education and when the patient will have recovered psychologically from the acute thromboembolic event

Answer Key

1. **Correct answer, (d)** While polymorphisms of factor V Leiden and the prothrombin gene mutation increase the risk of an initial VTE event, epidemiological studies have shown that mutations in these genes are not associated with recurrent events. However, unprovoked (idiopathic) VTE carries with it a high risk of recurrence, as high as 50 % over the 10 years following the index event.
2. **Correct answer, (c)** Thrombophilia testing is unlikely to impact the management plan in an elderly patient with a hip fracture or a patient with known malignancy. Thrombophilia testing is unlikely to be high-yield in a young patient with upper extremity DVT who most likely has Paget-Schroetter disease with upper extremity venous "effort" thrombosis due to repetitive motion in the setting of thoracic outlet compression. However, in the younger sister of a young woman with no other risk factors who develops DVT in the setting of starting an oral contraceptive pill, thrombophilia testing may impact the future decisions regarding the care of the patient and her family members.
3. **Correct answer, (c)** Assessment for the factor V Leiden mutation and the prothrombin gene mutation involves molecular genetic testing that is not impacted by the presence of acute thromboembolism or anticoagulation. Acute thromboembolism or anticoagulation can lower levels of protein C, protein S, and antithrombin resulting in the misdiagnosis of a factor deficiency. A normal or high level of protein C, protein S, or antithrombin in the setting of acute thromboembolism or anticoagulation does not correspond with a pathological state.

References

1. Piazza G. Thrombophilia testing, recurrent thrombosis, and women's health. Circulation. 2014;130:283–7.
2. Christiansen SC, Cannegieter SC, Koster T, Vandenbroucke JP, Rosendaal FR. Thrombophilia, clinical factors, and recurrent venous thrombotic events. JAMA. 2005;293:2352–61.

3. Lijfering WM, Middeldorp S, Veeger NJ, et al. Risk of recurrent venous thrombosis in homozygous carriers and double heterozygous carriers of factor V Leiden and prothrombin G20210A. Circulation. 2010;121:1706–12.
4. Goldhaber SZ, Grodstein F, Stampfer MJ, et al. A prospective study of risk factors for pulmonary embolism in women. JAMA. 1997;277:642–5.
5. Ageno W, Becattini C, Brighton T, Selby R, Kamphuisen PW. Cardiovascular risk factors and venous thromboembolism: a meta-analysis. Circulation. 2008;117:93–102.
6. Steffen LM, Folsom AR, Cushman M, Jacobs Jr DR, Rosamond WD. Greater fish, fruit, and vegetable intakes are related to lower incidence of venous thromboembolism: the Longitudinal Investigation of Thromboembolism Etiology. Circulation. 2007;115:188–95.
7. Rosengren A, Freden M, Hansson PO, Wilhelmsen L, Wedel H, Eriksson H. Psychosocial factors and venous thromboembolism: a long-term follow-up study of Swedish men. J Thromb Haemost. 2008;6:558–64.
8. Piazza G, Goldhaber SZ. Venous thromboembolism and atherothrombosis. Circulation. 2010;121:2146–50.
9. Piazza G, Goldhaber SZ, Lessard DM, Goldberg RJ, Emery C, Spencer FA. Venous thromboembolism in patients with symptomatic atherosclerosis. Thromb Haemost. 2011;106:1095–102.
10. Rogers MA, Levine DA, Blumberg N, Flanders SA, Chopra V, Langa KM. Triggers of hospitalization for venous thromboembolism. Circulation. 2012;125:2092–9.
11. Piazza G. Beyond Virchow's Triad: does cardiovascular inflammation explain the recurrent nature of venous thromboembolism? Vasc Med. 2015;20:102–4.
12. Folsom AR, Lutsey PL, Astor BC, Cushman M. C-reactive protein and venous thromboembolism. A prospective investigation in the ARIC cohort. Thromb Haemost. 2009;102:615–9.
13. Zee RY, Glynn RJ, Cheng S, Steiner L, Rose L, Ridker PM. An evaluation of candidate genes of inflammation and thrombosis in relation to the risk of venous thromboembolism: the Women's Genome Health Study. Circ Cardiovasc Genet. 2009;2:57–62.
14. Savchenko AS, Martinod K, Seidman MA, et al. Neutrophil extracellular traps form predominantly during the organizing stage of human venous thromboembolism development. J Thromb Haemost. 2014;12:860–70.
15. Glynn RJ, Danielson E, Fonseca FA, et al. A randomized trial of rosuvastatin in the prevention of venous thromboembolism. N Engl J Med. 2009;360:1851–61.
16. Piazza G, Goldhaber SZ, Lessard DM, Goldberg RJ, Emery C, Spencer FA. Venous thromboembolism in heart failure: preventable deaths during and after hospitalization. Am J Med. 2011;124:252–9.
17. Piazza G, Seddighzadeh A, Goldhaber SZ. Heart failure in patients with deep vein thrombosis. Am J Cardiol. 2008;101:1056–9.
18. Piazza G, Goldhaber SZ, Kroll A, Goldberg RJ, Emery C, Spencer FA. Venous thromboembolism in patients with chronic obstructive pulmonary disease. Am J Med. 2012;125:1010–8.

Chapter 3
Pathophysiology of Deep Vein Thrombosis and Pulmonary Embolism: Beyond Virchow's Triad

Abstract Deep vein thrombosis (DVT) and pulmonary embolism (PE) result from a combination of pathophysiological states including endothelial injury, stasis, inflammation, and hypercoagulability. The extent of the PE, the patient's underlying cardiopulmonary reserve, and compensatory neurohumoral adaptations determine the overall hemodynamic impact. The right ventricle (RV) plays a central role in PE pathophysiology. A sudden increase in RV afterload due to PE can lead to RV dilation and hypokinesis, RV ischemia, and ultimately acute RV failure.

Keywords Deep vein thrombosis • Pathophysiology • Pulmonary embolism • Right ventricle

Self-Assessment Questions

1. Which of the following processes result in increased pulmonary vascular resistance and RV pressure overload in the setting of acute PE?

   (a) Direct physical obstruction of the pulmonary arterial tree, hypoxemic vasoconstriction, and decreased RV cardiac output
   (b) Direct physical obstruction of the pulmonary arterial tree, hypoxemic vasoconstriction, and release of potent pulmonary arterial vasoconstrictors
   (c) Direct physical obstruction of the pulmonary arterial tree, right-to-left shunting through a patent foramen ovale, and release of potent pulmonary arterial vasoconstrictors
   (d) Direct physical obstruction of the pulmonary arterial tree, hypoxemic vasoconstriction, and interventricular septal deviation toward the RV

2. Hemodynamic collapse due to acute PE may occur as a result of all of the following processes except?

   (a) RV dilatation and hypokinesis
   (b) Impaired LV filling
   (c) RV ischemia and infarction
   (d) Tricuspid regurgitation

© Springer International Publishing Switzerland 2015   15
G. Piazza et al., *Handbook for Venous Thromboembolism*,
DOI 10.1007/978-3-319-20843-5_3

Clinical Vignette

A 41-year-old obese woman with recent hospitalization for Crohn's Disease presented with sudden onset dyspnea and pleuritic pain. Two days prior to presentation, she noted right calf discomfort. In the Emergency Department, she was noted to be tachycardic to 110 beats per minute, hypotensive with a blood pressure of 86/52 mmHg, and hypoxemic with a room air oxygen saturation of 88 %. An electrocardiogram was significant for sinus tachycardia. A contrast-enhanced chest CT demonstrated bilateral PE (Fig. 3.1) with right ventricular (RV) enlargement (Fig. 3.2). Venous ultrasound demonstrated right popliteal DVT.

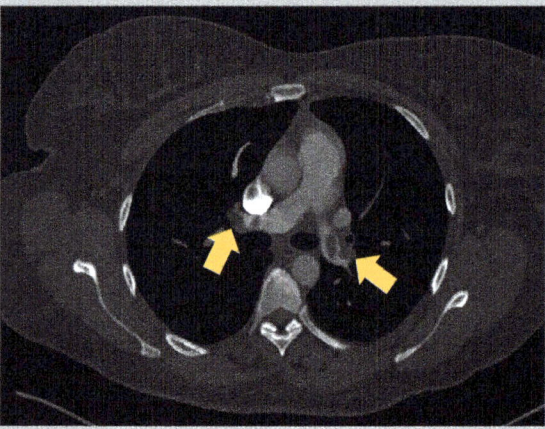

Fig. 3.1 Contrast-enhanced chest computed tomogram (CT) demonstrating bilateral pulmonary embolism (PE) (*arrows*) in a 41-year-old woman with dyspnea, pleuritic pain, and hypoxemia

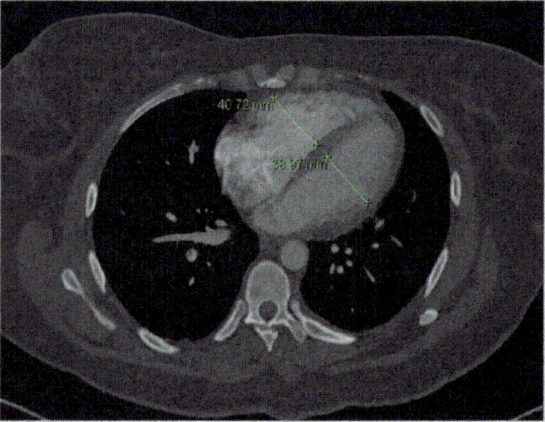

Fig. 3.2 Contrast-enhanced chest computed tomogram (CT) demonstrating right ventricular (RV) enlargement defined as an RV diameter-to-left ventricular diameter ratio greater than 0.9 in a 41-year-old woman with dyspnea, pleuritic pain, and hypoxemia who was diagnosed with bilateral pulmonary embolism (PE)

Pathophysiology of Deep Vein Thrombosis

Virchow's Triad of stasis, hypercoagulability, and endothelial dysfunction does not completely describe the pathophysiology of DVT in the majority of patients [1]. Immobility resulting in venous stasis is only a transient risk factor in most patients with VTE. Although frequently sought as an explanation for VTE, thrombophilia is diagnosed in only the minority of patients. The role of endothelial dysfunction in the pathophysiology of VTE remains poorly characterized. A growing body of literature suggests that cardiovascular inflammation is a key pathophysiologic factor in VTE. In epidemiologic analyses, systemic inflammation has been closely associated with an increased VTE risk. The increased frequency of DVT and PE in patients with chronic inflammatory disorders such as inflammatory bowel disease and systemic vasculitis highlights the pathophysiologic role of inflammation in VTE. Increased levels of the inflammatory biomarker C-reactive protein (CRP) augment VTE risk [2]. Integral components of the systemic inflammatory response, platelets and neutrophils, play a mechanistic role in the pathophysiology of VTE [3].

Although the deep veins of the lower extremity are the most common site for formation of DVT, thrombosis may also develop within the deep veins of the upper extremities, abdomen, and pelvis. May-Thurner Syndrome describes compression of the left common iliac vein by the right common iliac artery against the vertebral body and may result in extensive DVT of the left common iliac and distal venous segments. Cerebral venous thrombosis describes thrombosis of the cerebral veins and major dural sinuses [4].

Pathophysiology of Pulmonary Embolism

Most pulmonary emboli originate from the deep veins of the lower extremities and pelvis. The patient in the Clinical Vignette illustrates this observation because she was found to have right lower extremity DVT, the most likely source of her acute PE. Thrombi embolize from these veins and travel through the inferior vena cava (IVC), right atrium, and RV to lodge in the pulmonary arterial tree where they cause a variety of hemodynamic and gas exchange abnormalities.

The size of the embolus, the patient's underlying cardiopulmonary reserve, and compensatory neurohumoral adaptations determine the overall hemodynamic impact of PE [5]. Acute PE results in an abrupt increase in pulmonary vascular resistance and RV afterload through direct physical obstruction, hypoxemia, and release of pulmonary artery vasoconstrictors [6, 7]. The sudden increase in RV afterload can lead to RV dilation and hypokinesis, tricuspid regurgitation, and ultimately acute RV failure. Patients with RV failure may rapidly decompensate and develop systemic arterial hypotension, cardiogenic shock, and cardiac arrest. The patient in the Clinical Vignette illustrates the finding of RV failure due to acute PE with RV enlargement detected by chest CT and the development of systemic arterial hypotension. RV pressure overload can also result in diastolic interventricular septal

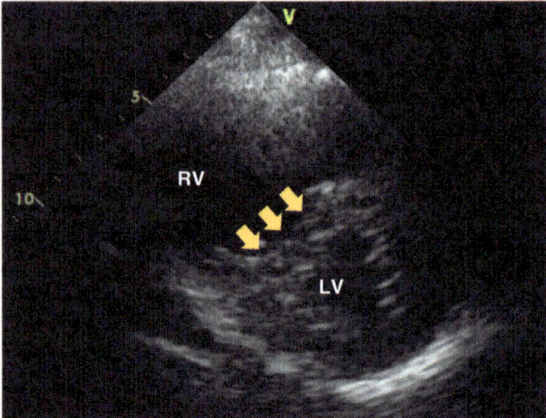

Fig. 3.3 Transthoracic echocardiogram, parasternal short axis view, demonstrating a markedly enlarged right ventricle (*RV*), underfilled left ventricle (*LV*), and interventricular septal deviation toward the LV (*arrows*) consistent with RV pressure overload in the setting of acute pulmonary embolism (PE)

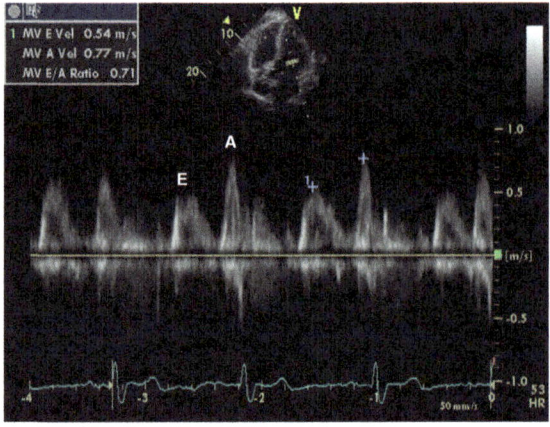

Fig. 3.4 Transthoracic echocardiogram, apical four-chamber view, transmitral Doppler flow pattern demonstrating left atrial contraction (*A* wave) making a greater contribution to left ventricular (LV) diastole than passive filling (*E* wave) consistent with LV diastolic impairment in a patient with right ventricular (RV) pressure overload in the setting of acute pulmonary embolism (PE)

deviation toward the left ventricle (LV), thereby impairing LV filling (Fig. 3.3). This phenomenon of interventricular dependence also leads to abnormal transmitral flow with left atrial contraction, represented by the A wave on Doppler echocardiography, making a greater contribution to LV diastole than passive filling, represented by the E wave (Fig. 3.4). RV pressure overload may also result in increased wall stress and ischemia by increasing myocardial oxygen demand while simultaneously limiting supply (Fig. 3.5).

Ventilation-to-perfusion mismatch, increases in total dead space, and right-to-left shunting contribute to the gas-exchange abnormalities observed in patients with

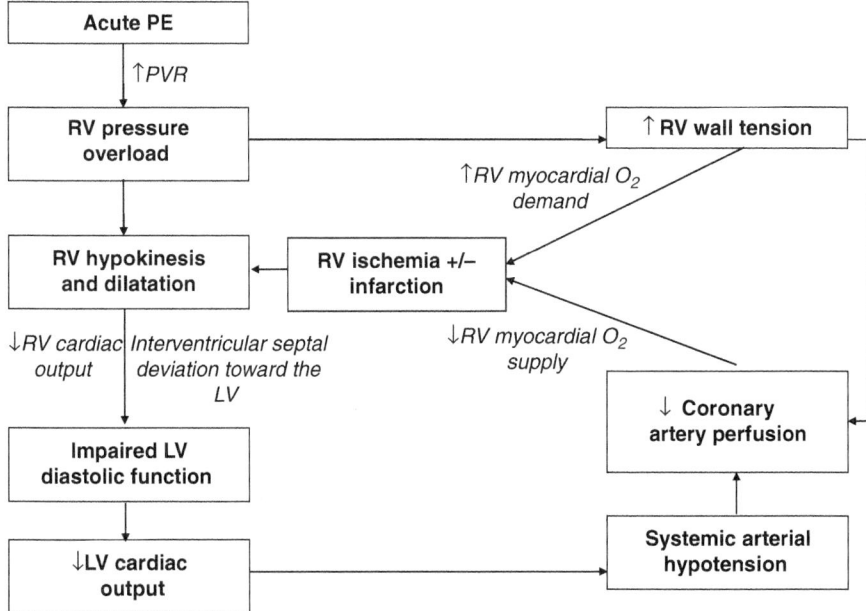

Fig. 3.5 The pathophysiology of right ventricular (*RV*) dysfunction due to acute pulmonary embolism (*PE*). *PVR* pulmonary vascular resistance, *LV* left ventricular

acute PE. The two most common abnormalities of gas exchange are arterial hypoxemia and increased alveolar-arterial oxygen gradient. Patients with acute PE may hyperventilate, leading to hypocapnia and respiratory alkalosis. Hypercapnia suggests massive PE, resulting in increased anatomic and physiological dead space and impaired minute ventilation.

Answer Key

1. **Correct answer**, (**b**) Acute PE results in an abrupt increase in pulmonary vascular resistance and RV afterload through direct physical obstruction, hypoxemia, and release of potent pulmonary artery vasoconstrictors. Decreased RV cardiac output and right-to-left shunting through a patent foramen ovale are the result of increased pulmonary vascular resistance rather than causes. Interventricular septal deviation toward the LV, not the RV, occurs in PE due to RV pressure overload.
2. **Correct answer**, (**d**) RV dilatation and hypokinesis, impaired LV filling, and RV ischemia and infarction can all result in hemodynamic collapse in the setting of acute PE. Although tricuspid regurgitation may result from an abrupt increase in pulmonary vascular resistance, it is rarely severe enough in the setting of acute PE to cause hemodynamic collapse.

References

1. Piazza G. Beyond Virchow's Triad: does cardiovascular inflammation explain the recurrent nature of venous thromboembolism? Vasc Med. 2015;20:102–4.
2. Folsom AR, Lutsey PL, Astor BC, Cushman M. C-reactive protein and venous thromboembolism. A prospective investigation in the ARIC cohort. Thromb Haemost. 2009;102:615–9.
3. Savchenko AS, Martinod K, Seidman MA, et al. Neutrophil extracellular traps form predominantly during the organizing stage of human venous thromboembolism development. J Thromb Haemost. 2014;12:860–70.
4. Piazza G. Cerebral venous thrombosis. Circulation. 2012;125:1704–9.
5. Piazza G. Submassive pulmonary embolism. JAMA. 2013;309:171–80.
6. Piazza G, Goldhaber SZ. The acutely decompensated right ventricle: pathways for diagnosis and management. Chest. 2005;128:1836–52.
7. Piazza G, Goldhaber SZ. Acute pulmonary embolism, Part I: Epidemiology and diagnosis. Circulation. 2006;114:e28–32.

Chapter 4
Diagnosis of Deep Vein Thrombosis: Incorporating Clinical Suspicion with Laboratory Testing and Imaging

Abstract Diagnosis of deep vein thrombosis (DVT) requires a high index of suspicion, especially in patients with venous thromboembolism (VTE) risk factors. A strategy that combines an assessment of clinical probability of the diagnosis with use of D-dimer testing and imaging when appropriate maximizes diagnostic accuracy. Venous ultrasound is the imaging test of choice for most patients with suspected DVT.

Keywords D-dimer • Deep vein thrombosis • Diagnosis • Ultrasound

Self-Assessment Questions

1. In which of the following patients would D-dimer testing for evaluation for suspected DVT be least likely to result in a false positive?

   (a) A 28-year-old man who presents to the Emergency Department with 2 days of right calf swelling, erythema, and tenderness
   (b) A 68-year-old woman who is 4 days status post left total knee replacement and reports left groin pain and thigh swelling
   (c) A 31-year-old woman who is 28 weeks pregnant and presents with asymmetric right ankle and calf edema
   (d) A 52-year-old man who is intubated in the Intensive Care Unit for treatment of acute respiratory distress syndrome (ARDS) in the setting of influenza infection who is noted to have left thigh and calf edema

2. Which of the following patients would be categorized as having a high probability of acute DVT according to the modified Wells Criteria?

   (a) A 67-year-old man with heart failure who presents to his primary care physician with bilateral ankle pitting edema after missing a few days of his diuretic therapy

© Springer International Publishing Switzerland 2015
G. Piazza et al., *Handbook for Venous Thromboembolism*,
DOI 10.1007/978-3-319-20843-5_4

(b) A 77-year-old man with prostate cancer status post prostatectomy 7 days prior who presents to the Emergency Department with complaint of left calf tenderness and swelling

(c) A 22-year-old collegiate women's basketball player who presents to the Student Health Center with right ankle pain and swelling and difficulty ambulating after a week of intensive pre-season practices

(d) A 69-year-old woman with alcoholic cirrhosis found bed-bound in her apartment and admitted with ascites, encephalopathy, and bilateral entire leg edema

3. In which of the following clinical scenarios would an alternative imaging technique such as CT, MR, or contract venography be appropriate?

(a) Evaluation of suspected DVT in a patient with a right upper extremity indwelling peripherally-inserted central catheter (PICC) and acute swelling of the right forearm and hand

(b) Evaluation of suspected DVT in a patient with left calf pain and swelling 1 week after left total knee replacement

(c) Evaluation of suspected DVT in a patient with left lower extremity edema and pain, a modified Wells score of 4, and a negative venous ultrasound

(d) Evaluation of suspected DVT in a patient with a history of PE status post insertion of an inferior vena cava filter who presents with right lower calf pain and ankle edema

Clinical Vignette

A 72-year-old man with a history of right lower extremity DVT following right ankle fracture 10 years prior and treated with anticoagulation for 6 months presented to the Emergency Department with sudden onset left leg discomfort and swelling. He had undergone cholecystectomy 2 weeks prior. Physical examination demonstrated slight redness, tenderness to palpation, and pitting edema of his left calf (Fig. 4.1). A venous ultrasound was performed and detected DVT in the left common femoral vein (Fig. 4.2).

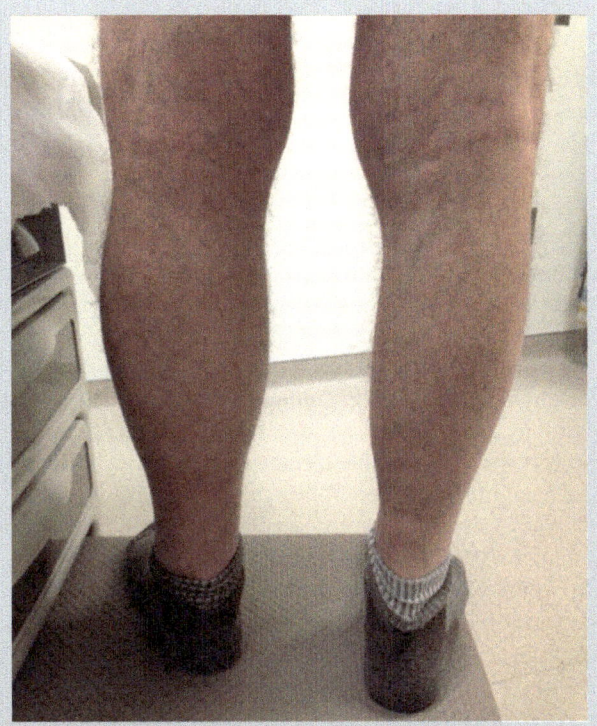

Fig. 4.1 Physical examination demonstrating slight redness and asymmetric swelling in a 72-year-old man with prior right-sided deep vein thrombosis (DVT) who presented with acute onset left calf pain and edema

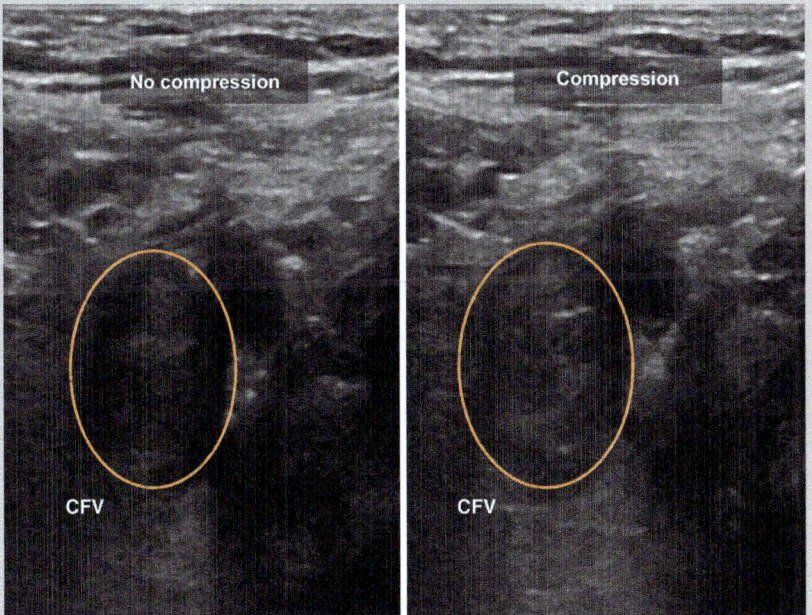

Fig. 4.2 Lower extremity venous ultrasound demonstrating a dilated and non-compressible left common femoral vein (*CFV*) (*ovals*) diagnostic of acute deep vein thrombosis (DVT) in a 72-year-old man with prior right-sided deep vein thrombosis (DVT) who presented with acute onset left calf pain and edema

Clinical Clues

Although it is most frequently observed in the lower extremities, DVT may also develop in the upper extremity veins in the setting of chronically indwelling central venous foreign bodies such as catheters or pacemakers, and syndromes of thoracic outlet obstruction [1, 2]. Patients with lower extremity DVT will commonly describe a cramping or pulling sensation of the lower calf that may worsen with ambulation. Warmth, edema, and tenderness of the lower extremity may be present on physical examination. Occasionally, a palpable cord or prominent venous collaterals may be appreciated. Importantly, some patients may not demonstrate any abnormalities on physical examination.

Alternative diagnoses to DVT include phlebitis without thrombosis, superficial vein thrombosis, venous insufficiency without acute thrombosis, post-thrombotic syndrome, ruptured Baker's cyst, muscle or soft tissue injury, hematoma, cellulitis, lymphedema, and peripheral edema secondary to congestive heart failure, liver disease, renal failure, or nephrotic syndrome (Table 4.1).

An assessment of pre-test probability guides the use of laboratory testing and imaging for the evaluation of DVT. Clinical decision rules organize clues from the history and physical examination and quantify the likelihood of DVT diagnosis. One such clinical decision rule, a modified version of the Wells clinical decision rule, assigns 1 point each for active cancer, recent surgery or immobility, paralysis, localized tenderness, entire leg swelling, calf swelling greater than 3 cm, pitting edema, collateral superficial veins, and subtracts 2 points for an alternative diagnosis as likely or greater than DVT (Table 4.2) [3]. DVT is high probability if the patient's score is greater than or equal to 3, moderate with a score of 1–2, and low if the score is 0 or less.

Table 4.1 Alternative diagnoses to deep vein thrombosis (DVT)	
	Phlebitis without thrombosis
	Superficial vein thrombosis
	Venous insufficiency without acute thrombosis
	Post-thrombotic syndrome
	Ruptured Baker's cyst
	Muscle or soft tissue injury
	Hematoma
	Cellulitis
	Lymphangitis
	Lymphedema
	Peripheral edema secondary to congestive heart failure
	Liver failure
	Renal failure
	Nephrotic syndrome
	Varicose veins

Table 4.2 A generally accepted clinical decision rule for the evaluation of patients with suspected deep vein thrombosis (DVT)

Variable	Points
Active cancer	1
Paralysis	1
Recently bedridden for >3 days or major surgery within 4 weeks	1
Localized tenderness along the distribution of the deep venous system	1
Entire leg swelling	1
Calf swelling >3 cm when compared with the asymptomatic leg[a]	1
Pitting edema	1
Collateral superficial veins (non-varicose)	1
Alternative diagnosis as likely or more likely than that of DVT	−2
"High Probability" ≥3 points	
"Moderate Probability" 1–2 points	
"Low Probability" ≤0 points	

[a]In patients with symptoms in both legs, the more symptomatic leg is used

Table 4.3 Common conditions that elevate D-dimer

Myocardial Infarction
Cancer
Pregnancy
Post-operative state
Infection
Liver disease
Renal disease
Eclampsia
Trauma
Aortic dissection

Laboratory Evaluation

D-dimer is a nonspecific marker of ineffective endogenous fibrinolysis and is elevated in VTE, including DVT, as well as other systemic illnesses and conditions such as surgery and pregnancy (Table 4.3). D-dimer is most useful in the evaluation of outpatients or Emergency Department patients with suspected VTE because inpatients will frequently have elevated levels secondary to other conditions. A systematic review of D-dimer studies in patients with suspected acute DVT demonstrated that the quantitative D-dimer enzyme-linked immunosorbent assay (ELISA) had negative likelihood ratios similar to those for negative venous duplex ultrasonography [4]. D-dimer for the evaluation of patients with suspected acute DVT offers the greatest accuracy when used in combination with an assessment of clinical probability [3]. In patients with low probability, a negative D-dimer can exclude the diagnosis of DVT without the need of further testing such as ultrasonography. Among patients with a high clinical suspicion for DVT, further diagnostic evaluation may be indicated despite negative D-dimer results.

Imaging Studies

Venous Ultrasound

Venous ultrasound is the initial imaging test of choice in the evaluation of suspected lower as well as upper extremity DVT. Venous ultrasound is superb for both the diagnosis and exclusion of an initial episode of DVT in both symptomatic and asymptomatic patients. Duplex venous ultrasound combines vein compression (B-mode imaging) and pulsed Doppler spectrum analysis with and without color. Failure to fully compress a vein ("non-compressibility") is diagnostic of DVT. Anatomic limitations hinder ultrasonographic evaluation of the pelvic veins and the upper extremity veins proximal to the clavicle.

Other Imaging Modalities

Alternative imaging modalities for assessment of patients with suspected acute DVT include CT, magnetic resonance (MR), and contrast venography. These imaging techniques are used when the evaluation by duplex venous ultrasound is inadequate or inconclusive. If a high clinical suspicion persists despite negative venous ultrasound or if acute-on-chronic thrombosis is suspected, MR, CT, or contrast venography may also be indicated. MR venography provides excellent resolution of the venous system, helps quantitate the precise clot burden, and is particularly useful for the evaluation of suspected pelvic vein or upper extremity DVT (Fig. 4.3). MR direct thrombus imaging is a sensitive and reproducible technique for distinguishing acute from chronic DVT and assessing changes in thrombus volume over time [5, 6].

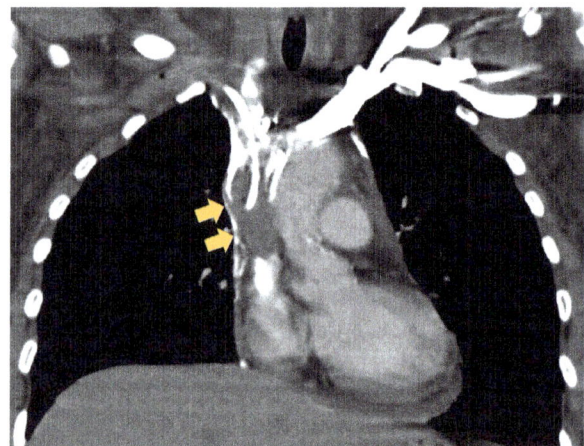

Fig. 4.3 Computed tomographic (CT) venography demonstrating superior vena cava (SVC) thrombosis (*arrows*) associated with an indwelling central venous catheter in a 54-year-old woman with bilateral upper extremity pain and edema admitted to the Intensive Care Unit with severe sepsis

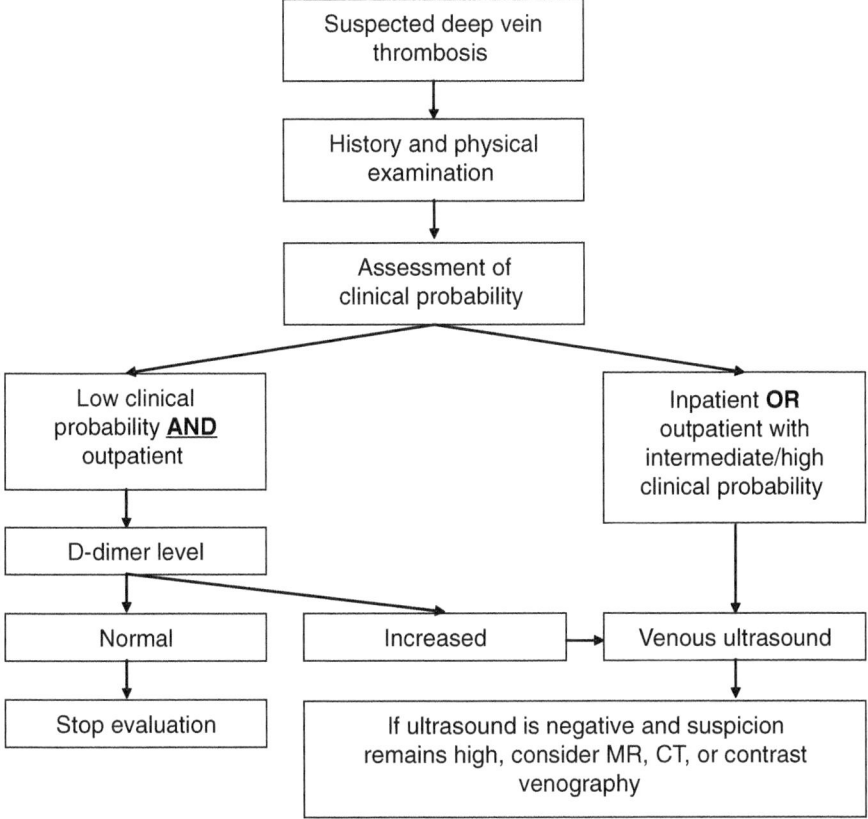

Fig. 4.4 Overall diagnostic algorithm for evaluation of suspected deep vein thrombosis (DVT). *MR* magnetic resonance, *CT* computed tomographic

Integrated Diagnostic Algorithm

An overall diagnostic algorithm for the evaluation of patients with suspected DVT integrates an assessment of clinical probability with D-dimer testing and diagnostic imaging (Fig. 4.4). The diagnosis of DVT can be excluded if there is low clinical probability and full compressibility on venous ultrasound. Of note, clinical decision rules validated for assessment of suspected DVT in outpatients may not be as useful among hospitalized patients [7].

The patient in the Clinical Vignette would be classified as high probability with a total point score of four based on one score point assigned for each clinical criterion of recent major surgery, lower extremity tenderness, asymmetric swelling, and pitting edema. Because a high clinical probability of acute DVT was present, D-dimer testing was not performed. Rather, the patient proceeded directly to venous ultrasound, which established the diagnosis of acute DVT.

Answer Key

1. **Correct answer**, (**a**) Recent surgery, pregnancy, and a systemic inflammatory response all increase D-dimer levels and complicate its use in the evaluation of patients with suspected DVT. D-dimer elevation in a young patient without other comorbid conditions and symptoms consistent with DVT is most likely to correspond with a true positive result.
2. **Correct answer**, (**b**) A high probability of DVT according to the modified Wells criteria corresponds with a score of 3 or higher. The 67-year-old man with heart failure would score 1 point for the finding of edema but would then lose 2 points because non-adherence to his diuretic regimen is a more likely cause of bilateral pitting edema than DVT. The 77-year-old man with prostate cancer has active malignancy, is post-operative, and has left calf tenderness and swelling yielding a score of 4 points. The 22-year-old women's basketball player and the 69-year-old woman with alcoholic cirrhosis both have other explanations for lower extremity symptoms that are more likely than DVT.
3. **Correct answer**, (**c**) CT, MR, and contrast venography are appropriate testing modalities for patients with a high suspicion of DVT despite an initially negative venous ultrasound. In such patients, DVT in a more proximal venous segment such as a pelvic vein may be missed by venous ultrasound due to anatomical constraints.

References

1. Joffe HV, Kucher N, Tapson VF, Goldhaber SZ. Upper-extremity deep vein thrombosis: a prospective registry of 592 patients. Circulation. 2004;110:1605–11.
2. Kucher N. Clinical practice. Deep-vein thrombosis of the upper extremities. N Engl J Med. 2011;364:861–9.
3. Wells PS, Owen C, Doucette S, Fergusson D, Tran H. Does this patient have deep vein thrombosis? JAMA. 2006;295:199–207.
4. Stein PD, Hull RD, Patel KC, et al. D-dimer for the exclusion of acute venous thrombosis and pulmonary embolism: a systematic review. Ann Intern Med. 2004;140:589–602.
5. Tan M, Mol GC, van Rooden CJ, et al. Magnetic resonance direct thrombus imaging differentiates acute recurrent ipsilateral deep vein thrombosis from residual thrombosis. Blood. 2014;124:623–7.
6. Westerbeek RE, Van Rooden CJ, Tan M, et al. Magnetic resonance direct thrombus imaging of the evolution of acute deep vein thrombosis of the leg. J Thromb Haemost. 2008;6:1087–92.
7. Silveira PC, Ip IK, Goldhaber SZ, Piazza G, Benson CB, Khorsani R. Wells score for deep vein thrombosis: performance in the inpatient setting. JAMA Intern Med. 2015;175:1112–7.

Chapter 5
Diagnosis of Pulmonary Embolism: An Integrated Approach to Clinical Evaluation, Laboratory Testing, and Imaging

Abstract Like deep vein thrombosis (DVT), a high clinical suspicion is required, especially in patients with venous thromboembolism (VTE) risk factors, to make a timely diagnosis of pulmonary embolism (PE). Diagnosis of acute PE is often challenging because the disease presents as a variety of clinical syndromes, ranging from pleuritic pain to cardiac arrest. A diagnostic algorithm that integrates an assessment of clinical probability with appropriate laboratory testing and imaging modalities is critical. Contrast-enhanced chest computed tomogram (CT) is the predominant imaging test used to diagnosis PE.

Keywords Chest CT • D-dimer • Diagnosis • Pulmonary embolism

Self-Assessment Questions

1. In which of the following clinical scenarios would D-dimer testing be an appropriate step in the evaluation of suspected acute PE?

   (a) A 23-year-old woman who recently started a combination oral contraceptive pill and presents to Urgent Care Clinic with acute dyspnea and pleuritic pain
   (b) A 68-year-old man with history of chronic obstructive pulmonary disease admitted to the Intensive Care Unit with severe community-acquired pneumonia requiring mechanical ventilation and progressive hypoxemia and new asymmetric left lower extremity edema
   (c) A 72-year-old woman with breast cancer status post mastectomy who recently started tamoxifen and now presents to the Emergency Department with hemoptysis and dyspnea
   (d) A 33-year-old man with recent Achilles tendon rupture status post recent repair who presents to his Primary Care Physician with pleuritic pain and dyspnea

2. Which of the following statements about imaging studies for evaluation of suspected acute PE is false?

   (a) Ventilation-perfusion lung scanning is generally reserved for patients with contraindications to iodinated contrast or ionizing radiation.
   (b) Advances in chest CT technology have increased the detection rate of subsegmental PE and have reduced the frequency of nondiagnostic studies.

© Springer International Publishing Switzerland 2015
G. Piazza et al., *Handbook for Venous Thromboembolism*,
DOI 10.1007/978-3-319-20843-5_5

  (c) Contrast pulmonary angiography is reserved for the circumstance in which noninvasive imaging modalities are nondiagnostic and a high clinical suspicion persists.
  (d) Bedside transthoracic echocardiography is sensitive for the diagnosis of acute PE in critically-ill patients who are unstable for transportation to the CT scanner.

3. Based on the results of the Christopher Study and Prospective Investigation of Pulmonary Embolism Diagnosis (PIOPED) II, what would be the most appropriate next step in a 45-year-old woman with suspected PE, a Wells score of 6, and a negative contrast-enhanced chest CT?

  (a) No further action is needed because the contrast-enhanced chest CT is negative.
  (b) Check a D-dimer test and perform additional imaging if positive.
  (c) Perform a transthoracic echocardiogram to evaluate for RV dysfunction as a surrogate for the diagnosis of PE.
  (d) Order a contrast pulmonary angiogram because a high suspicion for PE persists despite the negative chest CT.

Clinical Vignette
A 54-year-old obese woman with diabetes, hypertension, and hyperlipidemia presented to the Emergency Department with sudden onset dyspnea and chest pain. She denied any recent major surgery, trauma, or immobility. Upon physical examination, she was noted to have a heart rate of 96 beats per minute, blood pressure of 124/72 mmHg, and room air oxygen saturation of 85 %. Her electrocardiogram and chest X-ray were unremarkable. Her initial laboratory evaluation was normal except for an increased D-dimer result. Given her symptoms and positive D-dimer, she underwent a contrast-enhanced chest CT which demonstrated bilateral PE (Fig. 5.1).

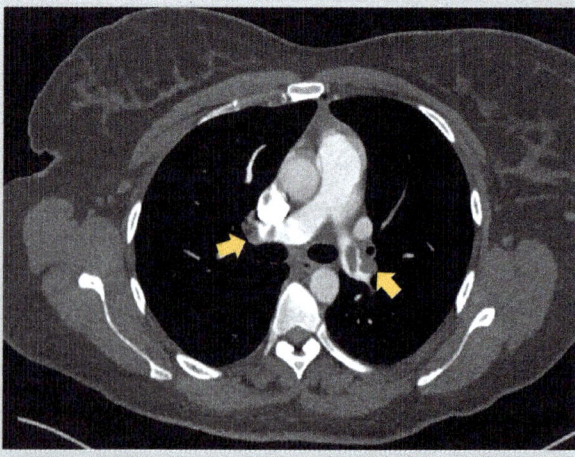

Fig. 5.1 Contrast-enhanced chest computed tomogram (CT) demonstrating bilateral pulmonary embolism (PE) (*arrows*) in a 54-year-old woman with dyspnea and chest pain

Clinical Clues

Acute PE can present with a wide spectrum of symptoms and signs. Dyspnea is the most frequently reported symptom. Severe dyspnea, cyanosis, or syncope suggests a massive PE, whereas pleuritic pain, cough, or hemoptysis may indicate a smaller peripherally located PE. Because acute coronary syndromes are so common and clinical suspicion is often high, clinicians may overlook the possibility of a life-threatening acute PE and inadvertently discharge these patients from the hospital after the exclusion of myocardial infarction with serial cardiac biomarkers and electrocardiograms.

On physical examination, tachypnea is the most common sign. Patients without underlying cardiopulmonary disease may appear anxious but well compensated, even with an anatomically extensive PE. Patients with massive PE may present with systemic arterial hypotension, cardiogenic shock, or cardiac arrest. Submassive PE describes patients who have preserved systolic blood pressure but exhibit evidence of RV failure such as tachycardia, distended neck veins, tricuspid regurgitation, and an accentuated sound of pulmonic closure (P2).

Alternative diagnoses to PE include acute coronary syndromes, exacerbations of chronic obstructive pulmonary disease, aortic dissection, pneumonia, acute bronchitis, decompensated heart failure, pulmonary hypertension, pericardial disease, musculoskeletal pain, pneumothorax, and hepatobiliary or splenic pathology, which may lead to referred pleuritic discomfort (Table 5.1).

Laboratory Evaluation

The laboratory evaluation of suspected acute PE should focus on the use of D-dimer testing in appropriately selected patients. Although it is nonspecific, D-dimer, as measured by enzyme-linked immunosorbent assay (ELISA), has utility in the evaluation of patients with suspected PE, especially in the Emergency Department

Table 5.1 Alternative diagnoses to acute pulmonary embolism (PE)	
	Acute coronary syndromes
	Chronic obstructive pulmonary disease exacerbation
	Aortic dissection
	Pneumonia
	Acute bronchitis
	Decompensated heart failure
	Pulmonary hypertension
	Pericardial disease
	Intrathoracic malignancy
	Musculoskeletal pain
	Pneumothorax
	Anxiety
	Hepatobiliary or splenic pathology

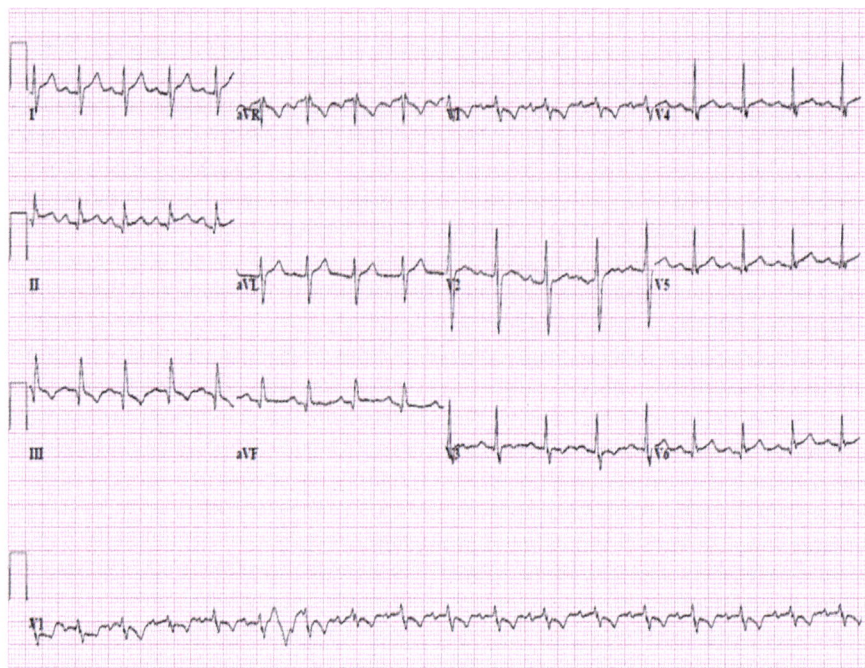

Fig. 5.2 12-lead electrocardiogram in a patient with acute pulmonary embolism (PE) demonstrating a deep S wave in Lead I, a deep Q wave in Lead III, and a T wave inversion in Lead III (S1Q3T3) consistent with right ventricular (RV) strain. The electrocardiogram also demonstrates sinus tachycardia, a common finding in patients with acute PE

setting. A study of patients with suspected acute PE in a high-volume Emergency Department demonstrated that the D-dimer ELISA had a sensitivity of 96.4 % and negative predictive value of 99.6 % [1]. Because of its high negative predictive value, the D-dimer ELISA can be used to exclude PE in outpatients with low to moderate pretest probability, without need for costly imaging and radiation exposure [2]. Most inpatients should proceed directly to an imaging study without D-dimer testing for PE because it is likely they will already have elevated D-dimers due to comorbid conditions.

Electrocardiogram

The electrocardiogram may reveal the presence of RV strain or may suggest concomitant or alternative diagnoses such as myocardial infarction or pericarditis (Fig. 5.2). Signs of RV strain secondary to PE include incomplete or complete right bundle branch block (RBBB), T wave inversions in the anterior precordium, as well as an S wave in lead I and a Q wave and T wave inversion in lead III (S1Q3T3) (Table 5.2). Some patients may only demonstrate signs of increased adrenergic

Table 5.2 Electrocardiographic findings in acute pulmonary embolism (PE)	Sinus Tachycardia
	Incomplete or complete right bundle branch block
	T wave inversions in leads III and aVF or in leads V1–V4
	S wave in lead I and a Q wave and T wave inversion in lead III (S1Q3T3)
	QRS axis greater than 90° or an indeterminate axis
	S waves in lead I and aVL greater than 1.5 mm
	Q waves in lead III and aVF, but not in lead II
	Transition zone shift toward V5
	Low voltage in the limb leads
	Atrial fibrillation

tone, with a resting sinus tachycardia. Furthermore, the electrocardiogram may be entirely normal, especially in young, previously healthy patients.

Imaging Studies

Chest X-Ray

Like the electrocardiogram, the chest X-ray serves an important role in detecting alternative or concomitant diagnoses such as pneumonia. A normal or near-normal chest X-ray in a patient with dyspnea or hypoxemia may suggest PE. However, the majority of patients with PE will have some abnormality such as cardiomegaly or pleural effusion on chest X-ray. Classic findings such as focal oligemia (Westermark sign), a peripheral wedge-shaped opacity (Hampton hump), or an enlarged right descending pulmonary artery (Palla's sign) are rare.

Chest Computed Tomography

Contrast-enhanced chest CT is the predominant diagnostic imaging technique for evaluation of suspected PE (Fig. 5.3). Advances in multi-detector array CT technology, from 16-, 64-, 128-, 256-, to 320-slice, have resulted in progressive improvements in spatial and temporal resolution [3]. The enhanced resolution of newer multi-detector CT scanners has increased the detection rate of subsegmental PE and has reduced the frequency of nondiagnostic studies when compared with older single-detector model [3]. An overview of chest CT in the assessment of patients with suspected acute PE demonstrated negative predictive values of 99.1 and 99.4 % for PE and PE-attributed mortality, respectively [4]. Based on these data, chest CT appears to be at least as accurate as invasive contrast pulmonary angiography.

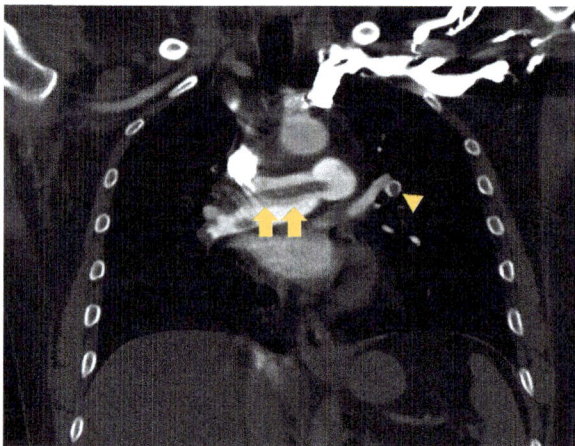

Fig. 5.3 Contrast-enhanced chest computed tomogram (CT) demonstrating a large "saddle" pulmonary embolism (PE) straddling the bifurcation of the pulmonary arterial trunk (*arrows*) in a 46-year-old man with profound dyspnea and cardiogenic shock. A smaller segmental PE (*arrowhead*) is noted in a segmental branch of the left pulmonary arterial tree

Ventilation-Perfusion Lung Scanning

Typically, ventilation-perfusion (V/Q) lung scans are reserved for patients with severe chronic kidney disease, anaphylaxis to intravenous iodinated contrast, or pregnancy (Fig. 5.4). Although a high probability scan in the setting of moderate to high clinical suspicion virtually guarantees the diagnosis and a normal scan excludes it, most patients have intermediate or indeterminate probability scans. Patients with nondiagnostic scans require further imaging to evaluate for PE.

Magnetic Resonance Angiography

Gadolinium-enhanced magnetic resonance (MR) angiography offers the benefit of avoiding the risks of iodinated contrast and ionizing radiation. However, gadolinium-based contrast is contraindicated in patients with acute kidney injury or chronic kidney disease with an estimated glomerular filtration rate <30 ml/min because of the risk of nephrogenic systemic fibrosis. MR angiography has shown limited sensitivity in the diagnosis of acute PE [5].

Echocardiography

Although insensitive for diagnosis, transthoracic echocardiography is a critical risk stratification tool for patients with proven acute PE. Echocardiography is superb for detecting RV dysfunction in the setting of PE with RV pressure overload (Fig. 5.5).

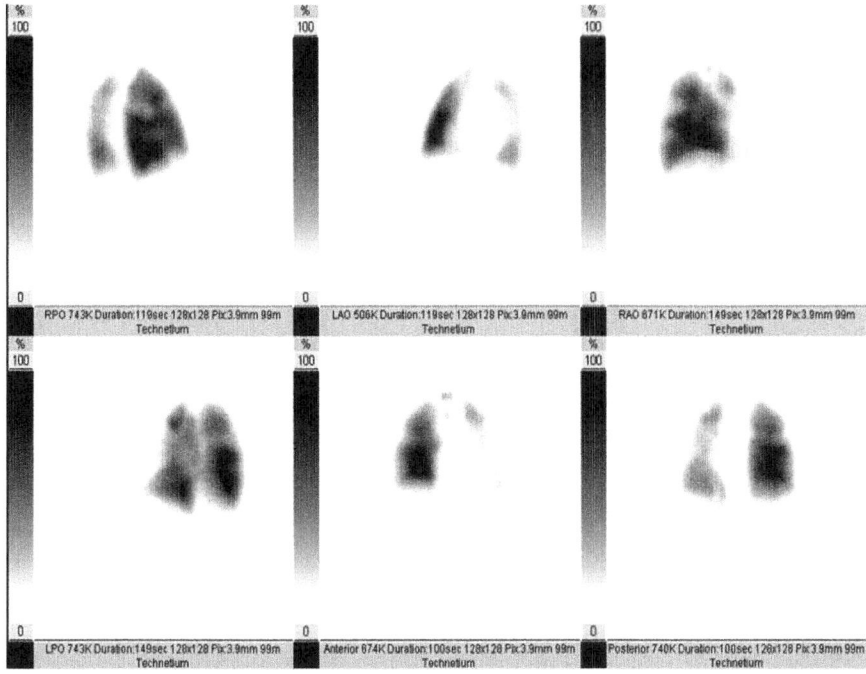

Fig. 5.4 Ventilation-perfusion lung scan, perfusion images, demonstrating multiple perfusion defects (*dark areas*) that were unmatched on the ventilation images diagnostic of acute pulmonary embolism (PE) in a 41-year-old woman with acute dyspnea and chest pain and history of anaphylaxis to iodinated contrast

Fig. 5.5 Transthoracic echocardiogram, apical four-chamber view, demonstrating a dilated right ventricle (*RV*) that is larger than the left ventricle (*LV*) in a 71-year-old man with acute pulmonary embolism (PE). Under normal conditions, RV end-diastolic diameter is no greater than 60 % of that of the LV

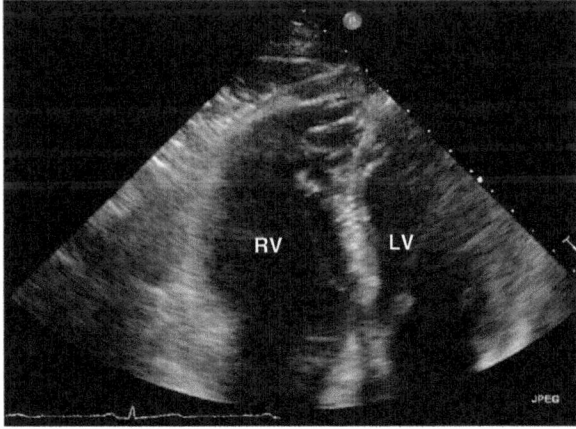

Typical echocardiographic findings among patients with acute PE include RV dilation and hypokinesis, paradoxical interventricular septal motion toward the LV, tricuspid regurgitation, and pulmonary hypertension as identified by a tricuspid regurgitant jet velocity greater than 2.6 m/s (Table 5.3) [6, 7]. Regional RV

Table 5.3 Echocardiographic findings in patients with acute pulmonary embolism (PE)

Right ventricular (RV) dilation and hypokinesis
Interventricular septal flattening and paradoxical motion toward the left ventricle (LV)
Increased RV diastolic diameter-to-LV diastolic diameter ratio
Tricuspid regurgitation
Pulmonary hypertension as identified by a tricuspid regurgitant jet velocity greater than 2.6 m/s
Dilation and loss of collapse of the inferior vena cava with inspiration
Decrease in the difference between LV area during diastole and systole (indicates low cardiac output state)
Decrease in tricuspid annular plane systolic excursion (TAPSE) <17 mm

dysfunction with severe free wall hypokinesis and apical sparing (McConnell sign) is a specific finding for PE [8]. Decreased tricuspid annular plane systolic excursion (TAPSE), which represents the distance of systolic excursion of the RV annular plane towards the apex (normal ≥17 mm), correlates with increased risk of PE-related death or need for fibrinolysis in patients with acute PE [9]. RV dysfunction is a clinically important echocardiographic finding among normotensive patients with acute PE because RV hypokinesis has been shown to be an independent risk predictor for early death [10]. In hemodynamically unstable patients, echocardiography can be performed rapidly at the bedside and may demonstrate evidence of RV failure suggestive of acute PE in addition to alternative diagnoses such as myocardial infarction, aortic dissection, and pericardial tamponade [11].

Transesophageal echocardiography may diagnose PE by direct visualization of the proximal pulmonary arteries. Transesophageal echocardiography is also useful in determining the extent of thrombus and surgical accessibility in patients being considered for surgical embolectomy [12].

Contrast Pulmonary Angiography

Contrast pulmonary angiography is reserved for the circumstance in which noninvasive imaging modalities are nondiagnostic and a high clinical suspicion persists. However, contrast pulmonary angiography is routinely employed when a catheter-directed therapeutic intervention is undertaken.

An Integrated Diagnostic Approach

A diagnostic algorithm that integrates an assessment of clinical probability with appropriate laboratory testing and imaging modalities is essential (Fig. 5.6). The Christopher Study employed an algorithm consisting of a dichotomized clinical decision rule using the Wells criteria, D-dimer testing, and chest CT to evaluate a

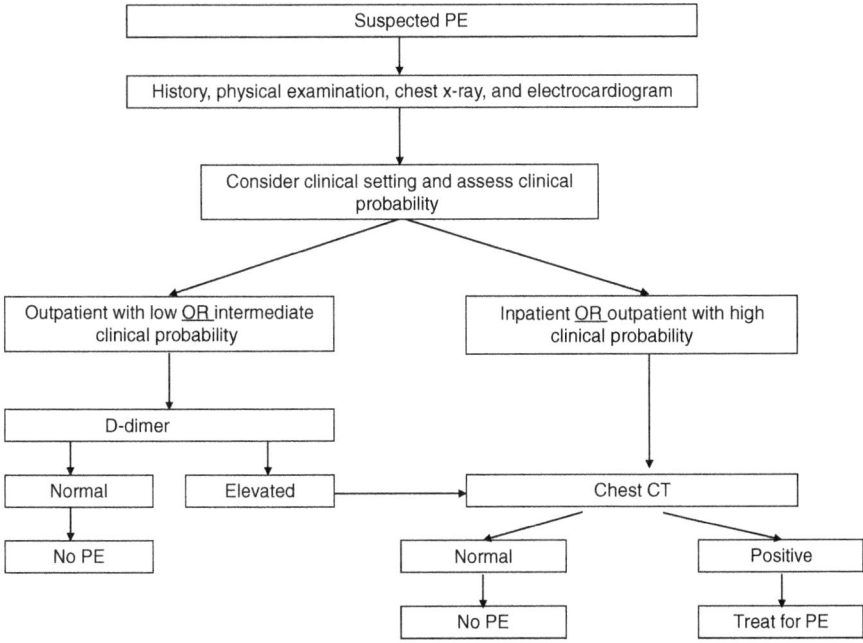

Fig. 5.6 An integrated diagnostic algorithm for patients with suspected pulmonary embolism (*PE*). *CT* computed tomography

cohort of patients with suspected acute PE [13]. The Wells criteria for clinical probability assessment assigns 3 points for clinical symptoms and signs of DVT, 3 points for an alternative diagnoses less likely than PE, 1.5 points for a heart rate greater than 100 beats per minute, 1.5 points for recent immobilization or surgery, 1.5 points for previous VTE, 1 point for hemoptysis, and 1 point for malignancy receiving treatment or palliative care within the last 6 months (Table 5.4). The patient illustrated in the Clinical Vignette would be assigned 3 points for an alternative diagnosis less likely that PE. Patients with 4 or less points are categorized as "PE unlikely" and those with greater than 4 points were classified as "PE likely." In the Christopher study, patients categorized as "PE likely" proceeded directly to chest CT. In contrast, patients classified as "PE unlikely" underwent D-dimer testing and were only referred for chest CT if the D-dimer level was abnormal. PE was considered to be excluded in patients classified as "PE unlikely" with negative D-dimer results and in patients with negative chest CT scans. This algorithm permitted a management decision in 98 % of patients and was associated with a low risk of VTE. The patient in the Clinical Vignette underwent D-dimer testing, the results of which were abnormal, and then chest CT, which confirmed the suspected PE.

The Prospective Investigation of Pulmonary Embolism Diagnosis II (PIOPED II) trial evaluated the accuracy of multidetector chest CT after assessment of the patient using a clinical decision rule [14]. Among patients with a low to intermediate clinical probability of acute PE, a negative chest CT had a high negative predictive value

Table 5.4 A generally accepted clinical decision rule for the evaluation of patients with suspected acute pulmonary embolism (PE)

Variable	Points
Clinical symptoms and signs of deep vein thrombosis (DVT)	3.0
Alternative diagnosis less likely than PE	3.0
Heart rate greater than 100 beats per minute	1.5
Recent immobilization or surgery	1.5
Previous venous thromboembolism	1.5
Hemoptysis	1.0
Malignancy receiving treatment or palliative care within the last 6 months	1.0
"PE unlikely" ≤4 points	
"PE likely" >4 points	

(96 % for patients with a low probability and 89 % for patients with an intermediate probability), whereas the negative predictive value was low (60 %) for patients with a high clinical probability [14, 15]. The addition of venous phase imaging of the lower extremities to chest CT added diagnostic sensitivity and modestly increased the negative predictive value when compared with chest CT alone [14, 15]. PIOPED II also suggested that additional testing may be necessary to confirm or exclude the diagnosis of PE when the clinical probability is discordant with the test results [14, 15]. MR angiography or invasive pulmonary angiography may be required to diagnose PE under these circumstances.

Both the Christopher Study and PIOPED II trial underscore the importance of an algorithm that integrates the use of a clinical decision rule with appropriate laboratory testing and imaging with chest CT. The use of such an algorithm facilitates management decisions and is associated with a low risk of VTE.

Answer Key

1. **Correct answer**, (**a**) D-dimer testing is likely to be abnormal in patients with acute infectious illness, active cancer, and recent surgery such that a positive result will be nonspecific for PE. Furthermore, patients with Wells scores >4 have a high clinical suspicion such that a negative D-dimer result should not terminate the evaluation for PE. A 23-year-old woman with a risk factor of oral contraceptive pill use and symptoms most consistent with PE would have a Wells score of 3. A normal D-dimer in this patient would have a high negative predictive value (>99 %), while an abnormal D-dimer would prompt further testing.

2. **Correct answer**, (**d**) Bedside transthoracic echocardiography is not sensitive for the diagnosis of acute PE. Transthoracic echocardiography is a critical risk stratification tool for patients with proven acute PE because it can rapidly and accurately

detect RV dysfunction. Transesophageal echocardiography may establish the diagnosis of PE by directly visualizing emboli in the proximal pulmonary arteries.

3. **Correct answer**, (**d**) PIOPED II suggested that additional imaging may be necessary to confirm or exclude the diagnosis of PE when the clinical probability is discordant with the test results. MR angiography or invasive pulmonary angiography is required to diagnose PE when the clinical suspicion is high but the chest CT has been interpreted as negative.

References

1. Dunn KL, Wolf JP, Dorfman DM, Fitzpatrick P, Baker JL, Goldhaber SZ. Normal D-dimer levels in emergency department patients suspected of acute pulmonary embolism. J Am Coll Cardiol. 2002;40:1475–8.
2. Stein PD, Hull RD, Patel KC, et al. D-dimer for the exclusion of acute venous thrombosis and pulmonary embolism: a systematic review. Ann Intern Med. 2004;140:589–602.
3. Hunsaker AR, Lu MT, Goldhaber SZ, Rybicki FJ. Imaging in acute pulmonary embolism with special clinical scenarios. Circ Cardiovasc Imaging. 2010;3:491–500.
4. Quiroz R, Kucher N, Zou KH, et al. Clinical validity of a negative computed tomography scan in patients with suspected pulmonary embolism: a systematic review. JAMA. 2005;293:2012–7.
5. Stein PD, Chenevert TL, Fowler SE, et al. Gadolinium-enhanced magnetic resonance angiography for pulmonary embolism: a multicenter prospective study (PIOPED III). Ann Intern Med. 2010;152:434–43.
6. Piazza G. Submassive pulmonary embolism. JAMA. 2013;309:171–80.
7. Piazza G, Goldhaber SZ. Management of submassive pulmonary embolism. Circulation. 2010;122:1124–9.
8. McConnell MV, Solomon SD, Rayan ME, Come PC, Goldhaber SZ, Lee RT. Regional right ventricular dysfunction detected by echocardiography in acute pulmonary embolism. Am J Cardiol. 1996;78:469–73.
9. Pruszczyk P, Goliszek S, Lichodziejewska B, et al. Prognostic value of echocardiography in normotensive patients with acute pulmonary embolism. JACC Cardiovasc Imaging. 2014;7:553–60.
10. Piazza G, Goldhaber SZ. Fibrinolysis for acute pulmonary embolism. Vasc Med. 2010;15:419–28.
11. Piazza G, Goldhaber SZ. The acutely decompensated right ventricle: pathways for diagnosis and management. Chest. 2005;128:1836–52.
12. Goldhaber SZ. Echocardiography in the management of pulmonary embolism. Ann Intern Med. 2002;136:691–700.
13. van Belle A, Buller HR, Huisman MV, et al. Effectiveness of managing suspected pulmonary embolism using an algorithm combining clinical probability, D-dimer testing, and computed tomography. JAMA. 2006;295:172–9.
14. Stein PD, Fowler SE, Goodman LR, et al. Multidetector computed tomography for acute pulmonary embolism. N Engl J Med. 2006;354:2317–27.
15. Perrier A, Bounameaux H. Accuracy or outcome in suspected pulmonary embolism. N Engl J Med. 2006;354:2383–5.

Chapter 6
Risk Stratification and Prognosis: Identifying Patients Who May Benefit from Advanced Therapies

Abstract A subset of initially normotensive patients with pulmonary embolism (PE) may clinically deteriorate and develop systemic arterial hypotension, cardiogenic shock, and sudden death, despite prompt therapeutic-level anticoagulation. Elevated cardiac biomarkers and right ventricular (RV) enlargement on imaging studies identify such vulnerable PE patients who may benefit from more advanced therapies. Clinical examination, electrocardiography, cardiac biomarker determination, chest computed tomogram (CT), and echocardiography are key instruments in the detection of RV dysfunction and risk stratification of patients with acute PE.

Keywords Cardiac biomarkers • Pulmonary embolism • Right ventricular dysfunction • Risk stratification

Self-Assessment Questions

1. All of the following predict increased risk of adverse outcomes in the setting of acute PE except?

   (a) A PE Severity Index (PESI) score of 55
   (b) Cardiac troponin elevation
   (c) Chest CT-measured RV diameter-to-LV diameter ratio greater than 0.9
   (d) RV dilation and hypokinesis detected by transthoracic echocardiography

2. Which of the following clinical parameters in the PESI is associated with the greatest incremental increase in risk?

   (a) Cancer
   (b) Systolic blood pressure <100 mmHg
   (c) Oxygen saturation <90 %
   (d) Abnormal mental status

3. Based on the 2014 European Society of Cardiology (ESC) Guidelines on the Diagnosis and Management of Acute Pulmonary Embolism, for which of the following patients would advanced therapy in addition to immediate anticoagulation be considered?

© Springer International Publishing Switzerland 2015   41
G. Piazza et al., *Handbook for Venous Thromboembolism*,
DOI 10.1007/978-3-319-20843-5_6

(a) A 23-year-old woman with acute PE, normal blood pressure and heart rate, hypoxemia with an oxygen saturation of 88 % on room air, normal cardiac troponin level, and chest CT-measured RV diameter-to-LV diameter ratio of 0.8.

(b) A 74-year-old man with acute PE, atrial fibrillation with a heart rate of 136 beats per minute, hypotension with a blood pressure of 82/58 mmHg, hypoxemia with an oxygen saturation of 84 % on room air, increased cardiac troponin, and a chest CT-measured RV diameter-to-LV diameter ratio of 1.2.

(c) A 66-year-old woman with acute PE, normal blood pressure, heart rate of 111 beats per minute, hypoxemia with an oxygen saturation of 89 % on room air, normal cardiac troponin level, and a transthoracic echocardiogram showing RV dilation and hypokinesis.

(d) A 70-year-old woman with acute PE, normal blood pressure, heart rate of 106 beats per minute, hypoxemia with an oxygen saturation of 87 % on room air, abnormal cardiac troponin level, and a transthoracic echocardiogram showing normal RV size and function.

Clinical Vignette

A 63-year-old man with hypertension, diabetes mellitus, and a recent rheumatoid arthritis exacerbation associated with relative immobility presented to the Emergency Department with sudden onset pleuritic pain, dyspnea at rest, and palpitations. Two days prior, he noted right lower extremity edema and pain upon ambulation which he attributed to rheumatoid arthritis. Upon physical examination, he was noted to have a heart rate of 112 beats per minute, blood pressure of 102/72 mmHg, respiratory rate of 24 breaths per minute, and room air oxygen saturation of 88 %. He has moderate pitting edema up to his right knee associated with erythema and tenderness to palpation along the calf. His electrocardiogram was remarkable for sinus tachycardia to 114 beats per minute. Given that a diagnosis of PE was "likely" (based on a Wells score of 9 points), he underwent a contrast-enhanced chest CT which demonstrated large bilateral PE (Fig. 6.1). The chest CT also documented RV enlargement as defined by an RV diameter-to-LV diameter ratio of 1.0 (Fig. 6.2). His initial laboratory evaluation was remarkable for a cardiac troponin of 0.4 ng/mL (normal range <0.01 ng/mL). Because of the elevated cardiac troponin, a bedside transthoracic echocardiogram was performed and demonstrated severe RV dilation and moderate pulmonary hypertension (Figs. 6.3 and 6.4).

Fig. 6.1 Contrast-enhanced chest computed tomogram (CT) demonstrating large bilateral pulmonary embolism (PE) (*arrows*) in a 63-year-old man with recent rheumatoid arthritis exacerbation associated with relative immobility and sudden onset pleuritic pain and dyspnea

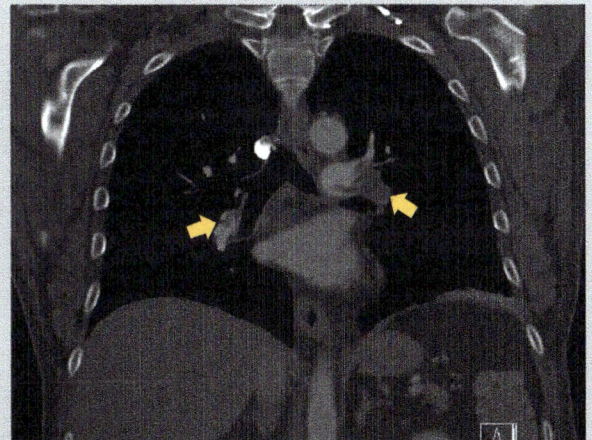

Fig. 6.2 Contrast-enhanced chest computed tomogram (CT) demonstrating right ventricular (RV) enlargement as defined by an increased RV diameter-to-left ventricular (LV) diameter ratio (3.82 cm/3.67 cm = 1.0; normal ≤0.9) in a 63-year-old man with acute pulmonary embolism (PE)

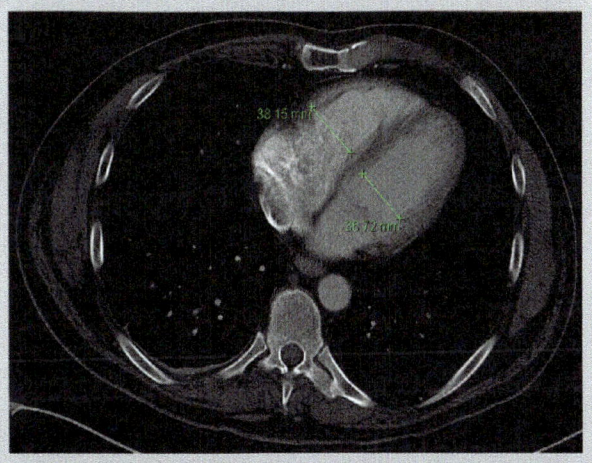

Fig. 6.3 Transthoracic echocardiogram, apical four-chamber view, demonstrating severe right ventricular (*RV*) dilatation relative to the left ventricle (*LV*) in a 63-year-old man with acute pulmonary embolism (PE)

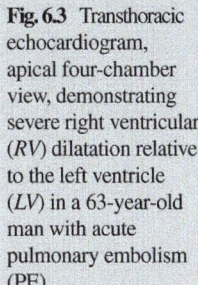

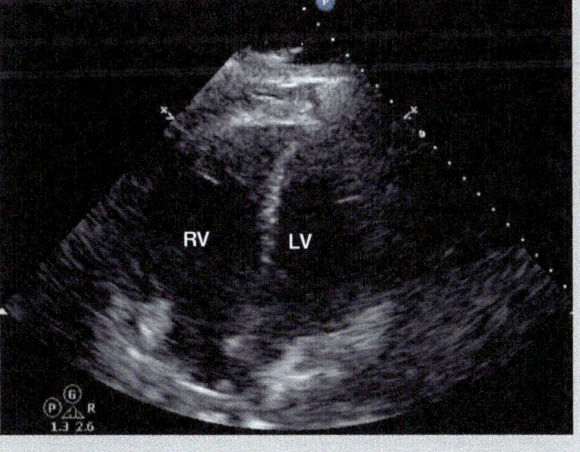

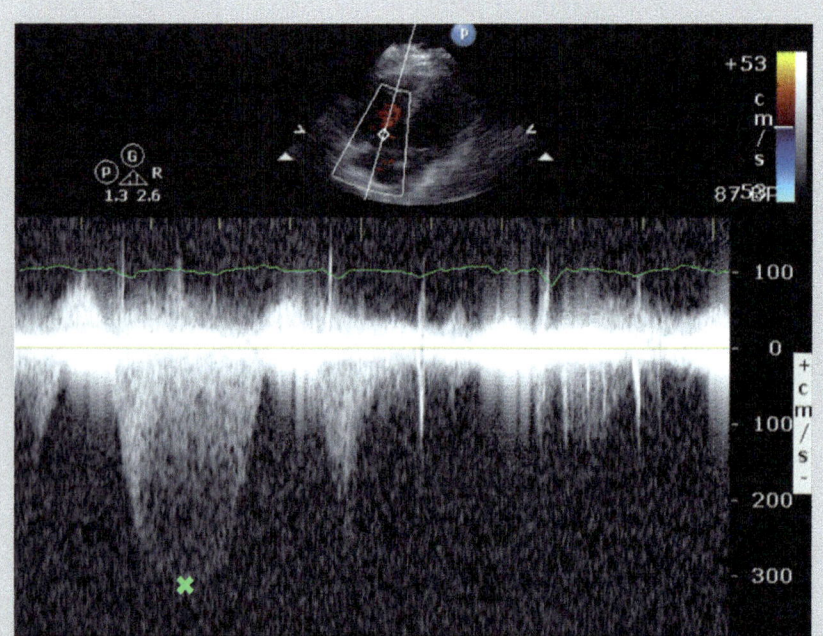

Fig. 6.4 Transthoracic echocardiogram, apical four-chamber view, demonstrating moderate pulmonary hypertension as defined by a peak tricuspid regurgitant jet velocity (X) of 300 cm/s in a 63-year-old man with acute pulmonary embolism (PE). Using the modified Bernoulli equation (4× [peak tricuspid regurgitant jet velocity]^2 + the estimate of right atrial pressure), the estimated pulmonary artery systolic pressure was 51 mmHg

Acute PE presents as a broad spectrum of clinical syndromes. Some patients complain of pleuritic pain, which usually results from small pulmonary emboli that affect nerve fibers in the periphery of the lung. In contrast, others may suffer massive PE resulting in syncope, systemic arterial hypotension, cardiogenic shock, or cardiac arrest. The majority of patients with acute PE presents with normal blood pressure. However, a subset of these initially normotensive patients may abruptly deteriorate and manifest systemic arterial hypotension, cardiogenic shock, and sudden death, despite prompt therapeutic-level anticoagulation. Accurate and rapid risk stratification to identify such vulnerable patients who may benefit from more advanced therapies has become a critical part of acute PE management. Clinical examination, electrocardiography, cardiac biomarker determination, chest CT, and echocardiography are key instruments in the detection of RV dysfunction and risk stratification of patients with acute PE.

Clinical Clues

The history and physical examination can provide important clues for risk stratification. The Pulmonary Embolism Severity Index (PESI) assigns 1 score point for the patient's age in years, 10 points for male sex, history of heart failure, and history of chronic lung disease, 20 points for a heart rate greater than or equal to 110 beats per minute, respiratory rate greater than or equal to 30 per minute, temperature less than 36 °C, and oxygen saturation less than 90 %, 30 points for history of cancer, and systolic blood pressure less than 100 mmHg, and 60 points for altered mental status (Table 6.1) [1, 2]. Patients with a score of 65 or less are classified as class I, or very low risk; 66–85 as class II, or low risk; 86–105 as class III, or intermediate risk; 106–125 as class IV, or high risk; and greater than 125 as class V, or very high risk. Class V corresponds with a class of patients at highest risk for 30-day mortality (25 %). In general, patients are not considered candidates for outpatient treatment of PE if their PESI score exceeds 85 points. A simplified PESI (sPESI) has also been evaluated and offers similar prognostic accuracy with greater ease of use [3]. The patient in the Clinical Vignette would be classified as high risk (Class IV) with a PESI point score of 113 (63 points for age + 10 points for male gender + 20 points for heart rate ≥100 beats per minute + 20 points for oxygen saturation <90 %).

Table 6.1 A generally accepted clinical decision rule for risk stratification of patients with acute pulmonary embolism (PE)

Variable	Points
Demographics	
Age, per year	Age, in years
Male sex	10
Comorbid illnesses	
History of cancer	30
History of heart failure	10
History of chronic lung disease	10
Clinical findings	
Heart rate ≥110 beats per minute	20
Systolic blood pressure <100 mmHg	30
Oxygen saturation <90 %[a]	20
Respiratory rate ≥30/min	20
Temperature <36 °C	20
Altered mental status[b]	60
Class I "very low risk" ≤65 points	
Class II "low risk" 66–85 points	
Class III "intermediate risk" 86–105 points	
Class IV "high risk" 106–125 points	
Class V "very high risk" >125 points	

[a]With and without the administration of supplemental oxygen
[b]Defined as disorientation, lethargy, stupor, or coma

Electrocardiography

The electrocardiogram is often one of the earliest indicators of RV dysfunction in the setting of acute PE [4]. In an analysis of the Management Strategies and Prognosis in Pulmonary Embolism Trial (MAPPET-1) registry, presence of any electrocardiographic abnormality (atrial arrhythmias, complete RBBB, low voltage in the limb leads, Q waves in leads III and aVF, or precordial ST segment changes) correlated with an increased risk of in-hospital mortality [5].

Cardiac Biomarkers

Elevations in cardiac biomarkers, including troponin, brain-type natriuretic peptide (BNP), and heart-type fatty acid-binding protein (H-FABP), are associated with RV dysfunction and are important tools for risk stratification [6]. RV pressure overload results in release of cardiac troponin due to RV microinfarction and secretion of BNP in response to increased RV shear stress [7]. Elevated levels of cardiac troponin and BNP are associated with increased short-term mortality and adverse outcomes in normotensive patients with acute PE [8, 9]. H-FABP, also released as a result of myocardial injury, diffuses more rapidly than troponin and is detectable earlier [10]. Patients with acute PE and normal H-FABP levels have an excellent prognosis regardless of echocardiographic findings, while those with increased levels of H-FABP have a higher rate of adverse events, even if echocardiography is normal [9]. The patient in the Clinical Vignette had an increased cardiac troponin consistent with myocardial necrosis due to RV pressure overload and increased risk of adverse clinical outcomes.

Imaging Studies

Chest Computed Tomography

Detection of RV enlargement by contrast enhanced chest CT is an especially convenient risk stratification tool because it utilizes data acquired from the initial diagnostic scan (Fig. 6.2). Based on measurements from an axial CT view, RV enlargement, defined as a ratio of RV diameter to LV diameter of greater than 0.9, has been found to be a significant independent predictor of mortality at 30 days [11–13]. A meta-analysis demonstrated that an increased RV diameter-to-LV diameter ratio correlated with at least a sevenfold increased risk of PE-related mortality [14]. RV diameter-to-LV diameter ratio serves as a surrogate for the RV volume-to-LV volume ratio. In the Clinical Vignette, the patient's RV diameter-to-LV diameter ratio of 1.0 identifies him as having increased risk of early mortality.

Echocardiography

Echocardiography is the best imaging study to detect RV dysfunction in the setting of acute PE and constitutes the core of risk stratification algorithms (Fig. 6.3). Normotensive patients with acute PE and evidence of RV dysfunction on echocardiography demonstrate an increased risk of systemic arterial hypotension, cardiogenic shock, and death, whereas those without RV dysfunction generally have a benign clinical course [15, 16]. Echocardiography should be performed in patients with acute PE and clinical evidence of RV failure, elevated cardiac biomarkers, suspected pulmonary arterial hypertension, clinical deterioration, or suspicion of other comorbid cardiac disease [17]. The addition of cardiac troponin levels to echocardiographic findings of RV dysfunction provides incremental information for risk stratification and helps to identify patients with a greater risk of PE-related death and all-cause mortality [18]. The patient in the Clinical Vignette had both evidence of RV dysfunction on transthoracic echocardiography and cardiac troponin elevation.

An Integrated Approach to Risk Stratification

Risk stratification in patients with acute DVT focuses on identifying those at increased risk for developing post-thrombotic syndrome which is characterized by chronic lower extremity pain, edema, and if advanced, venous ulceration. Patients with iliofemoral or femoral DVT have an increased risk of developing post-thrombotic syndrome and may benefit from advanced therapies such as catheter-directed fibrinolysis ("pharmacomechanical therapy") in addition to prompt anticoagulation [19]. Risk stratification for DVT dichotomizes patients into those with iliofemoral or femoral involvement and those with more distal disease (Fig. 6.5).

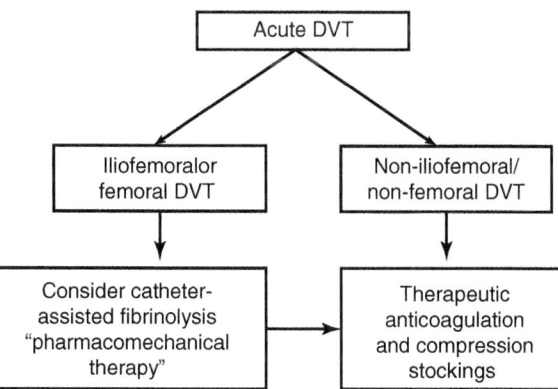

Fig. 6.5 An algorithm for risk stratification of patients with acute deep vein thrombosis (*DVT*)

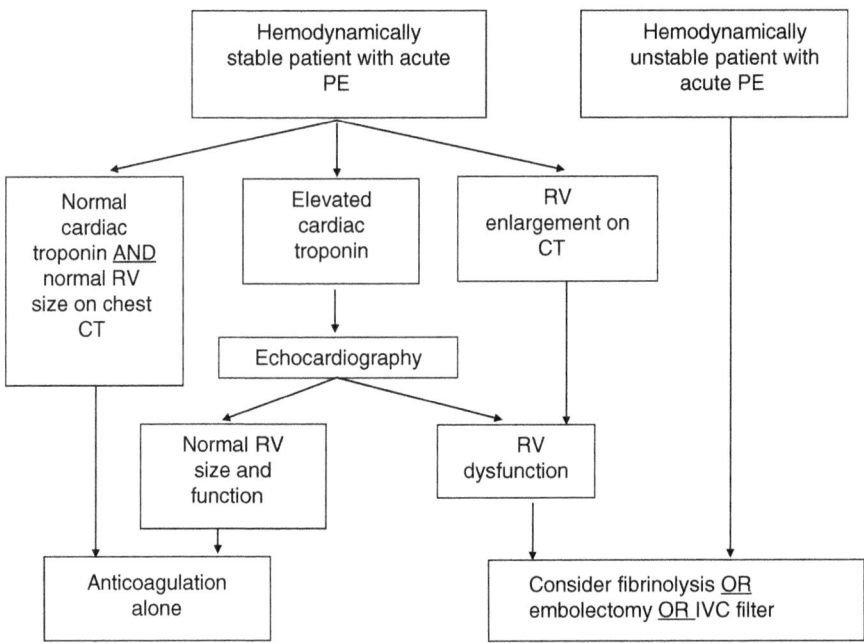

Fig. 6.6 An algorithm for risk stratification of patients with acute pulmonary embolism (*PE*). *RV* right ventricular, *CT* computed tomography, *IVC* inferior vena cava

For identification of patients with acute PE at risk for adverse outcomes, a risk stratification algorithm should integrate clinical prognostic indicators, cardiac biomarkers, and evidence of RV dysfunction as detected by either echocardiography or chest CT (Fig. 6.6) [20]. The 2014 European Society of Cardiology (ESC) Guidelines on the Diagnosis and Management of Acute Pulmonary Embolism emphasize the importance of an integrated approach for accurate identification of PE patients who are potential candidates for advanced therapy [21]. The 2014 ESC Guidelines classify patients into four categories of risk for early mortality: low, intermediate-low, intermediate-high, and high (Table 6.2). While low risk PE patients are characterized by preserved hemodynamics, a low PESI or Simplified PESI score, and no evidence of RV dysfunction or myocardial necrosis, high risk PE patients are marked by the presence of shock or hypotension. Intermediate-low risk PE patients are characterized by preserved hemodynamics but have an increased PESI or Simplified PESI score and either signs of RV dysfunction on imaging or elevated cardiac biomarkers (or neither). Intermediate-high risk PE patients also have preserved hemodynamics and an increased PESI or Simplified PESI score but have both signs of RV dysfunction on imaging and elevated cardiac biomarkers. High risk and intermediate-high risk PE patients are recommended to be considered for advanced therapies on a case-by-case basis. According to the 2014 ESC Guidelines, the patient in the Clinical Vignette would be categorized as intermediate-high risk for adverse clinical outcomes due to PE and would be considered for advanced therapy.

Table 6.2 2014 European Society of Cardiology (ESC) guidelines risk classification for patients with acute pulmonary embolism (PE)

Early mortality risk		Shock or hypotension	PESI class III-V or sPESI >1	RV dysfunction on imaging	Myocardial necrosis
High		Yes	Not required but "Yes" if assessed	Yes	Not required but "Yes" if assessed
Intermediate	Intermediate-high	No	Yes	Yes	Yes
	Intermediate-low	No	Yes	"Yes" for either one or neither	
Low		No	No	Not required but "No" if assessed	Not required but "No" if assessed

Answer Key

1. **Correct answer**, (**a**) A PE Severity Index (PESI) score ≤65 (Class I) corresponds with a very low risk of adverse events.
2. **Correct answer**, (**d**) Abnormal mental status contributes 60 score points in the PESI. Cancer, systolic blood pressure <100 mmHg, and oxygen saturation <90 % contribute 30 points, 30 points, and 20 points, respectively.
3. **Correct answer**, (**b**) The 74-year-old man with acute PE had systemic arterial hypotension, RV dysfunction on imaging, and elevated cardiac biomarkers (increased troponin) and would be classified as high risk per the 2014 ESC Guidelines. Only intermediate-high and high risk patients are considered for advanced therapy to treat acute PE.

References

1. Aujesky D, Obrosky DS, Stone RA, et al. Derivation and validation of a prognostic model for pulmonary embolism. Am J Respir Crit Care Med. 2005;172:1041–6.
2. Aujesky D, Roy PM, Le Manach CP, et al. Validation of a model to predict adverse outcomes in patients with pulmonary embolism. Eur Heart J. 2006;27:476–81.
3. Jimenez D, Aujesky D, Moores L, et al. Simplification of the pulmonary embolism severity index for prognostication in patients with acute symptomatic pulmonary embolism. Arch Intern Med. 2010;170:1383–9.
4. Geibel A, Zehender M, Kasper W, Olschewski M, Klima C, Konstantinides SV. Prognostic value of the ECG on admission in patients with acute major pulmonary embolism. Eur Respir J. 2005;25:843–8.
5. Kasper W, Konstantinides S, Geibel A, et al. Management strategies and determinants of outcome in acute major pulmonary embolism: results of a multicenter registry. J Am Coll Cardiol. 1997;30:1165–71.
6. Piazza G, Goldhaber SZ. Fibrinolysis for acute pulmonary embolism. Vasc Med. 2010;15: 419–28.

7. Kucher N, Goldhaber SZ. Cardiac biomarkers for risk stratification of patients with acute pulmonary embolism. Circulation. 2003;108:2191–4.
8. Becattini C, Vedovati MC, Agnelli G. Prognostic value of troponins in acute pulmonary embolism: a meta-analysis. Circulation. 2007;116:427–33.
9. Pieralli F, Olivotto I, Vanni S, et al. Usefulness of bedside testing for brain natriuretic peptide to identify right ventricular dysfunction and outcome in normotensive patients with acute pulmonary embolism. Am J Cardiol. 2006;97:1386–90.
10. Puls M, Dellas C, Lankeit M, et al. Heart-type fatty acid-binding protein permits early risk stratification of pulmonary embolism. Eur Heart J. 2007;28:224–9.
11. Dellas C, Puls M, Lankeit M, et al. Elevated heart-type fatty acid-binding protein levels on admission predict an adverse outcome in normotensive patients with acute pulmonary embolism. J Am Coll Cardiol. 2010;55:2150–7.
12. Schoepf UJ, Kucher N, Kipfmueller F, Quiroz R, Costello P, Goldhaber SZ. Right ventricular enlargement on chest computed tomography: a predictor of early death in acute pulmonary embolism. Circulation. 2004;110:3276–80.
13. van der Meer RW, Pattynama PM, van Strijen MJ, et al. Right ventricular dysfunction and pulmonary obstruction index at helical CT: prediction of clinical outcome during 3-month follow-up in patients with acute pulmonary embolism. Radiology. 2005;235:798–803.
14. Trujillo-Santos J, den Exter PL, Gomez V, et al. Computed tomography-assessed right ventricular dysfunction and risk stratification of patients with acute non-massive pulmonary embolism: systematic review and meta-analysis. J Thromb Haemost. 2013;11:1823–32.
15. Goldhaber SZ. Echocardiography in the management of pulmonary embolism. Ann Intern Med. 2002;136:691–700.
16. Kucher N, Rossi E, De Rosa M, Goldhaber SZ. Prognostic role of echocardiography among patients with acute pulmonary embolism and a systolic arterial pressure of 90 mm Hg or higher. Arch Intern Med. 2005;165:1777–81.
17. Piazza G, Goldhaber SZ. The acutely decompensated right ventricle: pathways for diagnosis and management. Chest. 2005;128:1836–52.
18. Stein PD, Matta F, Janjua M, Yaekoub AY, Jaweesh F, Alrifai A. Outcome in stable patients with acute pulmonary embolism who had right ventricular enlargement and/or elevated levels of troponin I. Am J Cardiol. 2010;106:558–63.
19. Kahn SR, Comerota AJ, Cushman M, et al. The postthrombotic syndrome: evidence-based prevention, diagnosis, and treatment strategies: a scientific statement from the American Heart Association. Circulation. 2014;130:1636–61.
20. Piazza G. Submassive pulmonary embolism. JAMA. 2013;309:171–80.
21. Konstantinides SV, Torbicki A, Agnelli G, et al. 2014 ESC Guidelines on the diagnosis and management of acute pulmonary embolism: the Task Force for the Diagnosis and Management of Acute Pulmonary Embolism of the European Society of Cardiology (ESC) Endorsed by the European Respiratory Society (ERS). Eur Heart J. 2014;35:3033–73.

Chapter 7
Advanced Therapy for Venous Thromboembolism: Understanding the Role of Systemic Fibrinolysis, Catheter-Based Therapy, and Surgery

Abstract Selection of patients with venous thromboembolism (VTE) for advanced therapies requires recognition of high-risk deep vein thrombosis (DVT) and pulmonary embolism (PE) syndromes. Advanced therapies for acute PE include systemic fibrinolysis, catheter-based "pharmacomechanical" intervention, and surgical pulmonary embolectomy. Choosing a particular advanced therapy depends on the individual patient's risk for adverse outcomes due to VTE and for major bleeding, specifically intracranial hemorrhage. Multidisciplinary PE Response Teams may facilitate access to advanced therapies and appropriate patient selection.

Keywords Catheter-based intervention • Deep vein thrombosis • Fibrinolysis • Pulmonary embolism • Surgical embolectomy • Therapy

Self-Assessment Questions

1. Which of the following statements regarding systemic fibrinolysis for acute PE is correct?

    (a) Compared with anticoagulation alone, systemic fibrinolysis reduces mortality only in patients with massive PE.
    (b) Compared with anticoagulation alone, systemic fibrinolysis reduces mortality in patients with massive and submassive PE at the cost of increased risk of intracranial hemorrhage.
    (c) Compared with anticoagulation alone, systemic fibrinolysis for acute PE reduces the risk of hemodynamic collapse but does not impact mortality.
    (d) Compared with anticoagulation alone, systemic fibrinolysis reduces the risk of recurrent PE and shortens length of stay but does not improve mortality.

2. Which of the following advanced therapies would be most appropriate in a 55-year-old man with acute dyspnea, tachycardia, and hypotension requiring vasopressor support who is diagnosed with "saddle" PE 1 week following laparotomy for small bowel obstruction?

(a) Full-dose systemic fibrinolysis
(b) Half-dose systemic fibrinolysis
(c) Surgical pulmonary embolectomy
(d) Inferior vena cava (IVC) filter insertion

Clinical Vignette

A 57-year-old obese man with severe three-vessel coronary artery disease status post coronary artery bypass graft surgery 5 years prior and history of heart failure with a left ventricular (LV) ejection fraction of 40–45 % presented to the Emergency Department with 5 days of progressive exertional dyspnea and an episode of syncope. Earlier in the week, the patient had seen his Primary Care Physician who increased his outpatient diuretic regimen. On the morning of presentation, he was walking to the bathroom when he felt lightheaded and then lost consciousness. On physical examination, he was tachycardic to 124 beats per minute, hypotensive with a blood pressure of 86/48 mmHg, and profoundly hypoxemic with an oxygen saturation of 94 % on a non-rebreather mask. His electrocardiogram was remarkable for sinus tachycardia. His chest X-ray demonstrated cardiomegaly without pulmonary edema. Contrast-enhanced chest computed tomogram (CT) demonstrated a large "saddle" PE (Fig. 7.1) and right ventricular (RV) enlargement with an RV diameter-to-LV diameter ratio of 1.3 (Fig. 7.2). Upon return from Radiology, the patient developed worsening hypoxemia and hypotension requiring bolus intravenous fluids. An urgent transesophageal echocardiogram demonstrated RV dilation, hypokinesis, and pressure overload (Fig. 7.3) and PE in the proximal pulmonary trunk (Fig. 7.4). The hospital PE Response Team was activated, and representatives from Pulmonary Medicine, Cardiovascular Medicine, and Cardiac Surgery convened at the bedside. After a consensus decision was made, the patient was administered recombinant tissue-plasminogen activator (t-PA) 100 mg via peripheral IV over 2 h with prompt improvement in oxygenation and hemodynamics.

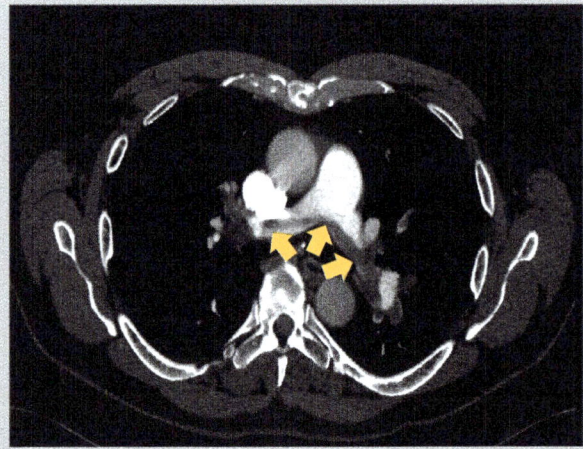

Fig. 7.1 Contrast-enhanced chest computed tomogram (CT) demonstrating large "saddle" pulmonary embolism (PE) (*arrows*) in a 57-year-old man with dyspnea on exertion and syncope

Fig. 7.2 Contrast-enhanced chest computed tomogram (CT) demonstrating right ventricular (RV) enlargement as defined by an increased RV diameter-to-left ventricular (LV) diameter ratio (4.9 cm/3.8 cm = 1.3; normal ≤ 0.9) in a 57-year-old man with acute pulmonary embolism (PE)

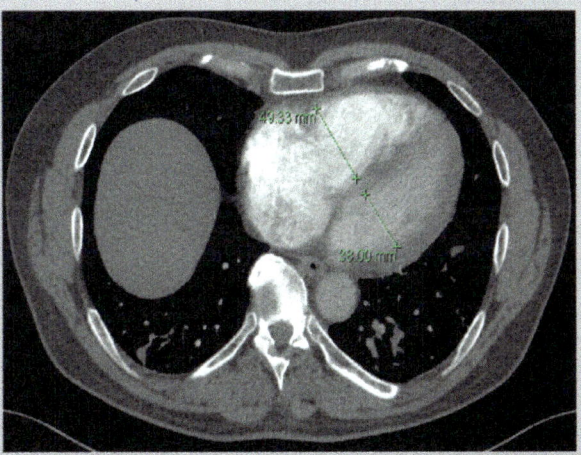

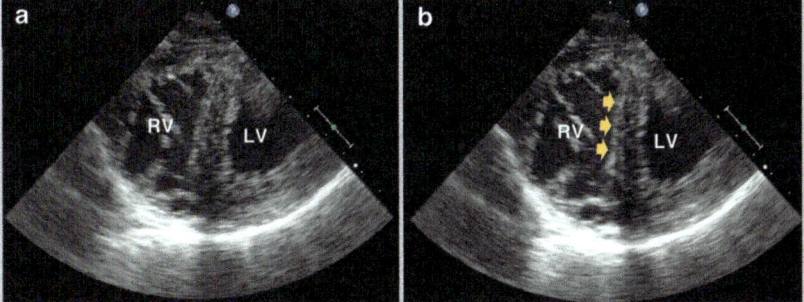

Fig. 7.3 Transesophageal echocardiogram, transgastric view, demonstrating right ventricular (*RV*) dilation in diastole with an underfilled left ventricle (*LV*) (panel **a**) in a 57-year-old man with acute pulmonary embolism (PE) and hypotension. In systole, the interventricular septum deviated toward the LV (*arrows*) consistent with RV pressure overload (panel **b**)

Fig. 7.4 Transesophageal echocardiogram demonstrating pulmonary embolism (PE) (*arrows*) in the proximal pulmonary trunk in a 57-year-old man with acute pulmonary embolism (PE) and hypotension

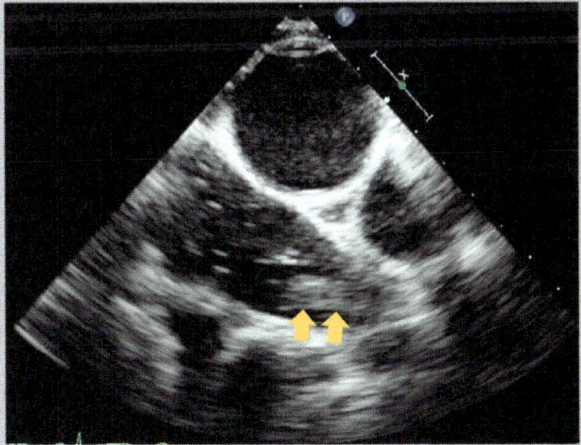

Spectrum of Disease

Deep Vein Thrombosis

DVT describes a wide spectrum of conditions, including massive DVT, proximal lower extremity DVT, isolated calf DVT, and upper extremity DVT.

Massive Deep Vein Thrombosis

Massive DVT most often describes thrombus that originates in the proximal veins of the lower extremity and extends into the iliac veins. Such extensive thrombus may result in severe post-thrombotic syndrome if not treated with advanced therapies such as pharmacomechanical catheter-directed fibrinolysis or thrombectomy.

Proximal Lower Extremity Deep Vein Thrombosis

Proximal DVT is the most common type of DVT and generally describes thrombus involving the common femoral, proximal femoral, distal femoral, or popliteal veins.

Isolated Calf Deep Vein Thrombosis

The previous practice of serial diagnostic testing with lower extremity ultrasound has been largely replaced by routine anticoagulation of symptomatic, isolated calf DVT. Patients with isolated calf DVT are at elevated risk for proximal propagation of the thrombus as well as for development of PE. Calf veins include the gastrocnemius, soleal, peroneal, posterior tibial, and anterior tibial veins. A proportion of patients will have duplicated venous segments that can contribute to underdiagnosis of DVT if the duplicated vein is not imaged.

Upper Extremity Deep Vein Thrombosis

Upper extremity DVT most often affects the subclavian, internal jugular, axillary, and brachial veins as a result of chronic indwelling foreign bodies such as central venous catheters and pacemaker or defibrillator leads [1]. Superior vena cava syndrome may complicate an upper extremity DVT secondary to venous foreign bodies or may result from thoracic malignancy with extrinsic compression of the upper extremity veins. Catheter-based fibrinolytic therapy is recommended for patients with acute proximal upper extremity DVT and severe symptoms, low risk for bleeding, and good functional status [2].

Pelvic Vein Thrombosis

Pelvic vein thrombosis describes DVT of the inferior vena cava (IVC), gonadal veins, and common, internal, and external iliac veins.

Mesenteric Vein Thrombosis

Mesenteric vein thrombosis describes DVT of the superior mesenteric vein most commonly but may also involve the inferior mesenteric vein, splenic vein, and portal veins [3].

Cerebral Venous Thrombosis

Cerebral venous thrombosis, including thrombosis of cerebral veins and major dural sinuses, is an uncommon disorder in the general population. However, it has a higher frequency among patients younger than 40 years old, patients with hypercoagulable states, and women who are pregnant or receiving hormonal contraceptive therapy [4].

Pulmonary Embolism

Acute PE describes a number of clinical syndromes, including massive PE, submassive PE, and PE with normal blood pressure and preserved RV function.

Massive Pulmonary Embolism

Massive PE accounts for approximately 5–10 % of cases and describes a subset of patients with PE who present with syncope, systemic arterial hypotension, cardiogenic shock, or cardiac arrest. The patient in the Clinical Vignette would be categorized as having massive PE because of his syncope and systemic arterial hypotension on presentation.

Submassive Pulmonary Embolism

Normotensive patients with acute PE and evidence of RV dysfunction are classified as having submassive PE and account for approximately 20–25 % of cases. These patients represent a population at increased risk of adverse events and early mortality [5].

Pulmonary Embolism with Normal Blood Pressure and Preserved Right Ventricular Function

Patients with acute PE presenting with normal systemic blood pressure and no evidence of RV dysfunction represent the majority of PE patients (approximately 70 %) and generally have a benign course when treated with standard anticoagulation alone.

Advanced Therapy

Fibrinolysis

Deep Vein Thrombosis

Fibrinolysis plus mechanical disruption of thrombus should provide a greater chance of preserving venous valve patency and function, thereby preventing chronic venous disease including post-thrombotic syndrome. Fibrinolytic therapy should be catheter-directed rather than peripherally-administered in DVT to gain access to the obstructed deep venous system [6].

Pulmonary Embolism

Advanced therapy with systemic fibrinolysis is reserved for patients presenting with either massive or submassive acute PE. The rationale for systemic fibrinolysis administered through a peripheral vein is to rapidly reverse hemodynamic compromise, RV dysfunction, and gas exchange abnormalities. Fibrinolytic therapy reverses systemic arterial hypotension by alleviating RV pressure overload [7]. In patients with submassive PE, fibrinolysis is administered to avert impending hemodynamic collapse and death from progressive right-sided heart failure. Systemic fibrinolysis may also function as a "medical embolectomy" that reduces thrombus burden, pulmonary vascular resistance, and RV dysfunction [8–10], and improves pulmonary capillary blood flow and gas exchange [11]. Finally, systemic fibrinolysis may help prevent the development of chronic thromboembolic pulmonary hypertension [12, 13] by preserving the normal hemodynamic response to exercise [14].

Fibrinolysis is usually considered a lifesaving therapy in patients presenting with massive PE [15–17]. The 2012 American College of Chest Physicians (ACCP) Evidence-Based Clinical Practice Guidelines on Antithrombotic Therapy for Venous Thromboembolism Disease suggest restricting the use of systemic fibrinolysis in submassive PE to a subset of these patients with a low risk of bleeding and a clinician-determined high risk of developing hemodynamic collapse (Grade 2C) [16]. The American Heart Association (AHA) Scientific Statement on Management of Massive and Submassive PE, Iliofemoral DVT, and Chronic Thromboembolic Pulmonary Hypertension recommends considering systemic fibrinolysis for submassive PE patients deemed to have evidence of adverse prognosis (new hemodynamic instability, worsening respiratory insufficiency, severe right ventricular dysfunction, or major myocardial necrosis) and a low risk of bleeding (Class IIb; Level of Evidence C) [15]. The 2014 European Society of Cardiology (ESC) Guidelines on the Diagnosis and Management of Acute Pulmonary Embolism recommend systemic fibrinolysis for PE with shock or hypotension (high-risk) (Class of Recommendation I, Level of Evidence B) [17]. The 2014 ESC Guidelines state that fibrinolytic therapy should be considered for patients with intermediate-high risk PE and clinical signs of hemodynamic decompensation (Class of Recommendation IIa, Level of Evidence B).

The Europe-based Pulmonary Embolism International Thrombolysis Trial (PEITHO) is the largest randomized controlled trial of systemic fibrinolysis in submassive PE to date, enrolling 1,006 submassive PE patients. The study evaluated the impact of systemic fibrinolysis with tenecteplase followed by anticoagulation with heparin versus heparin alone on the primary outcome of all-cause mortality or hemodynamic collapse within 7 days of randomization [18]. Fibrinolysis reduced the frequency of the primary outcome (2.6 % vs. 5.6 %, p=0.015) with the majority of the benefit due to a reduction in hemodynamic collapse within 7 days of randomization (1.6 % vs. 5 %, p=0.002). However, the benefit of fibrinolysis came at the cost of increased major bleeding (6.3 % vs. 1.5 %, p<0.001). More than 2 % of the tenecteplase-treated patients suffered intracranial hemorrhage, compared with 0.2 % in the heparin alone group.

Meta-analyses of trials of systemic fibrinolysis for acute PE have demonstrated both important benefits and critical limitations [19, 20]. Chatterjee and colleagues compared 1061 patients treated with fibrinolytic therapy with 1054 patients treated with anticoagulation alone [19]. Fibrinolytic therapy was associated with a reduction in all-cause mortality (2.2 % vs. 3.9 %; adjusted odds ratio [OR], 0.53; 95 % confidence interval, 0.32–0.88) and recurrent PE (1.2 % vs. 3.0 %; adjusted OR, 0.40; 95 % confidence interval, 0.22–0.74) compared with anticoagulation alone, resulting in a number needed to treat of 59 patients. The reduction in all-cause mortality with fibrinolytic therapy was sustained even when the meta-analysis was restricted to patients with submassive PE. Similar to the findings of PEITHO, the benefit of systemic fibrinolysis was offset by an increase in major bleeding (9.2 % versus 3.4 %; adjusted OR, 2.73; 95 % confidence interval, 1.91–3.91) in particular intracranial hemorrhage (1.5 % versus 0.2 %; adjusted OR, 4.78; 95 % confidence interval, 1.78–12.04).

Another meta-analysis by Marti and colleagues confirmed the finding of a reduction in all-cause mortality with fibrinolytic therapy for acute PE (adjusted OR, 0.59; 95 % confidence interval, 0.36–0.96) [20]. However, increased major bleeding (adjusted OR, 2.91; 95 % confidence interval, 1.95–4.36) and fatal or intracranial hemorrhage (adjusted OR, 3.18; 95 % confidence interval, 1.25–8.11) limited the benefit of fibrinolysis. Concern over the risk of intracranial hemorrhage, which approaches 3–5 % outside of clinical trials [21, 22], has dampened clinician enthusiasm for full-dose systemic fibrinolysis and has sparked development of alternative fibrinolytic strategies with lower bleeding risk.

One such alternative strategy focuses on half-dose systemic fibrinolysis [13, 23]. In the Moderate Pulmonary Embolism Treated with Thrombolysis (MOPETT) trial,

121 hemodynamically stable patients with acute symptomatic and anatomically large PE were randomized to either half-dose fibrinolysis with t-PA and concomitant anticoagulation versus standard anticoagulation with enoxaparin or heparin [13]. The frequency of pulmonary hypertension at 28 months was lower in patients who received fibrinolytic therapy than in the standard anticoagulation group (16 % vs. 57 %, p<0.001). No in-hospital bleeding events were reported in either study group. Mean length of hospital stay was decreased in those assigned to the fibrinolytic arm compared with standard anticoagulation (2.2 days vs. 4.9 days, p<0.001).

Administration

The U.S. Food and Drug Administration (FDA) has approved 100 mg t-PA (alteplase) as a continuous infusion over 2 h for the fibrinolysis of massive PE. Patients being considered for fibrinolysis should be meticulously assessed for contraindications (Table 7.1). In contrast to fibrinolysis in myocardial infarction, intravenous unfractionated heparin is withheld during the infusion of t-PA. The activated partial thromboplastin time (aPTT) should be checked immediately at the conclusion of the fibrinolytic infusion. Unfractionated heparin infusion should be restarted without a bolus as long as the aPTT is less than or equal to 80 s, which is the case most of the time. If still greater than 80 s, the aPTT should be rechecked every 4 h until it is less than 80 s. Then, heparin can be safely restarted. Although the efficacy of fibrinolytic therapy in PE appears to be inversely proportional to the duration of symptoms, effective fibrinolysis can be administered up to 2 weeks after an acute PE [24].

Surgical Interventions

Surgical thrombectomy is reserved for patients with massive or severely symptomatic DVT in whom fibrinolytic therapy is contraindicated or has failed. Surgical pulmonary embolectomy may be considered in patients with massive or submassive

Table 7.1 Major contraindications to fibrinolytic administration in pulmonary embolism (PE)	
	Intracranial mass
	Cerebrovascular event or neurosurgery within the prior 2 months
	History of intracranial hemorrhage
	Recent major trauma
	Active or recent respiratory, gastrointestinal, or genitourinary tract bleeding
	Severe uncontrolled hypertension
	Thrombocytopenia (<100,000 platelets/μL)
	Acute pericarditis or pericardial effusion
	Ongoing suspicion for aortic dissection
	Recent surgery, invasive procedure, or internal organ biopsy

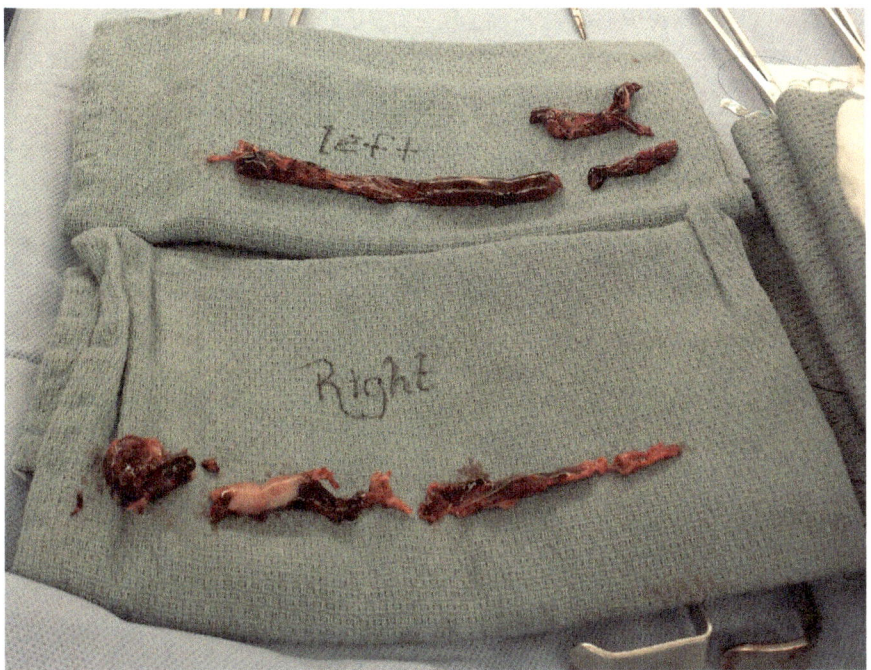

Fig. 7.5 Surgical pulmonary embolectomy specimen removed from a patient with massive pulmonary embolism (PE) (Image courtesy of Dr. Marzia Leacche)

PE in whom fibrinolysis has failed or is contraindicated. Rescue surgical pulmonary embolectomy after failed fibrinolysis is preferred over repeat administration of fibrinolytic therapy because of a lower rate of in-hospital adverse events [25]. Other indications include paradoxical embolism, persistent right heart thrombi, "clot-in-transit," and hemodynamic or respiratory compromise requiring cardiopulmonary resuscitation. Surgical pulmonary embolectomy is most effective in patients with large centrally-located PE. In specialized centers experienced in surgical pulmonary embolectomy, this operation has been shown to be safe and effective (Fig. 7.5) [26, 27]. To optimize results, refer the patient for surgery prior to the development of pressor-dependent hypotension and prior to the onset of multisystem organ failure.

Catheter-Assisted Pharmacomechanical Therapy

Catheter-assisted techniques for advanced therapy in both DVT and PE are most effective when combining pharmacological dissolution of the thrombus with local administration of fibrinolytic agent and mechanical disruption of the thrombus (called "pharmacomechanical therapy"). Catheter-assisted techniques combining local fibrinolysis with mechanical thrombectomy offer the potential advantage of increased efficacy of thrombus dissolution due to the synergistic effects of higher local fibrinolytic drug concentrations and facilitated drug penetration into the thrombus via mechanical disruption. Because higher local drug concentration is achieved with lower overall dose of fibrinolytic agent, catheter-directed therapy may offer the advantage of decreased hemorrhagic complications.

Catheter-assisted thrombectomy in DVT has historically been used most commonly to treat upper extremity thrombosis or iliofemoral DVT in patients with severe symptoms. In the CaVenT study, 209 patients with first-time iliofemoral DVT were randomized to standard anticoagulation alone or in combination with catheter-directed fibrinolysis. Co-primary endpoints were frequency of post-thrombotic syndrome as assessed by Villalta score at 24 months and iliofemoral patency after 6 months [28]. At 24 months, the frequency of post-thrombotic syndrome was reduced in patients who underwent catheter-directed fibrinolysis compared with those assigned to standard anticoagulation alone (41.1 % vs. 55.6 %, p=0.047). The difference in post-thrombotic syndrome correlated with a 14.4 % absolute risk reduction and a number-needed-to-treat of seven. Iliofemoral patency after 6 months was observed in 65.9 % of patients treated with catheter-directed fibrinolysis compared with 47.4 % of patients in the control group (p=0.012). Three major and five clinically-relevant nonmajor bleeds were reported in the catheter-directed fibrinolysis group compared with no reported bleeds in the standard anticoagulation group. The National Heart Lung and Blood Institute (NHLBI)-sponsored ATTRACT Trial (ClinicalTrials.gov Identifier: NCT00790335) has completed enrollment and will determine if catheter-based fibrinolytic therapy can safely prevent post-thrombotic syndrome and improve quality of life in patients with acute iliofemoral or femoral DVT.

Catheter-assisted techniques are considered for advanced therapy of acute PE when full-dose systemic fibrinolysis is contraindicated. Catheter-directed techniques are most successful when applied to large, centrally-located thrombi within the first 2 weeks of symptoms. Catheter-based pulmonary embolectomy is an emerging technique for advanced therapy in acute PE [29]. Several catheter-directed techniques are currently under investigation for treatment of acute PE. Catheter-directed ultrasound-facilitated low-dose fibrinolysis represents one emerging type of pharmacomechanical therapy in acute PE [30, 31].

In a European randomized controlled trial of 59 patients with submassive PE, ultrasound-facilitated, catheter-directed low-dose t-PA (20 mg total) plus anticoagulation reduced the RV diameter-to-LV diameter ratio from baseline to 24 h to a greater extent than anticoagulation alone [30]. In a U.S. single-arm, multicenter trial, the safety and efficacy of ultrasound-facilitated catheter-directed low-dose fibrinolysis was evaluated in 150 patients with acute massive (N=31) or submassive (N=119) PE [31]. Eligible patients were required to have proximal PE and RV diameter-to-LV diameter ratio of at least 0.9 on chest CT. Patients received a novel dose of tissue-plasminogen activator (t-PA): 24 mg administered either as 1 mg/h for 24 h with a unilateral catheter or 1 mg/h/catheter for 12 h with bilateral catheters. The primary safety outcome was major bleeding within 72 h of procedure initiation. The primary efficacy outcome was the change in chest CT-measured RV diameter-to-LV diameter

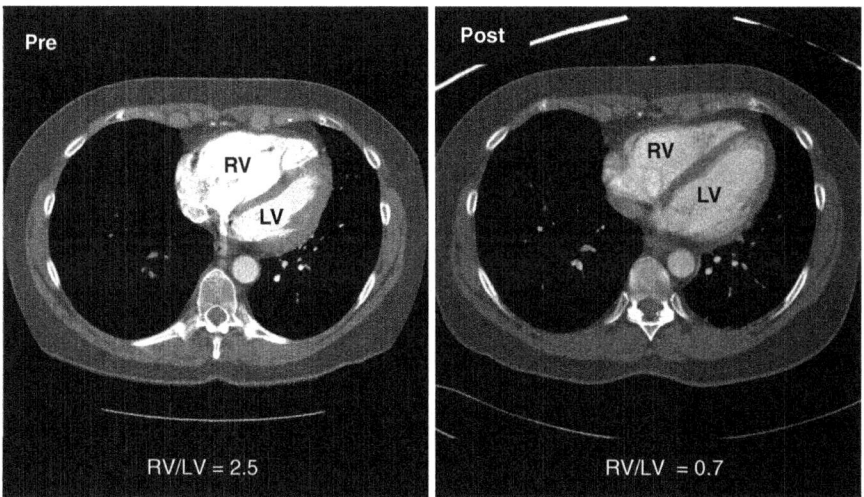

Fig. 7.6 Contrast-enhanced chest computed tomogram (CT) demonstrating rapid reduction in right ventricular (*RV*) diameter-to-left ventricular (*LV*) diameter ratio from pre-procedure to post-ultrasound-facilitated catheter-directed low-dose fibrinolysis in a patient with submassive pulmonary embolism (PE) (Images courtesy of Dr. Keith Sterling)

ratio within 48 h of procedure initiation. Mean RV diameter-to-LV diameter ratio improved by 25 % from pre- and at 48 h post-procedure (1.55 vs. 1.13; mean difference, −0.42; p < 0.0001) (Fig. 7.6). Mean pulmonary artery systolic pressure (51.4 mmHg vs. 36.9 mmHg; p < 0.0001) and modified Miller index (22.5 vs. 15.8; p < 0.0001) each improved by 30 % post-procedure. One GUSTO-defined severe bleed (groin hematoma with transient hypotension) and 16 GUSTO-defined moderate bleeding events occurred in 15 patients (10 %). No patient suffered intracranial hemorrhage. Based on these data, ultrasound-facilitated catheter-directed low-dose fibrinolysis appeared to be safe and effective. On May 21, 2014, the U.S. FDA approved ultrasound-facilitated, catheter-directed low-dose fibrinolysis with the EkoSonic® Endovascular System for treatment of PE.

Because many patients with acute PE have contraindications to fibrinolytic therapy, most often due to bleeding risk, catheter-assisted embolectomy without locally-administered fibrinolysis has been considered to be a promising alternative. However, in a systematic review of 594 acute PE patients, the pooled frequency of success (defined as stabilization of hemodynamics, resolution of hypoxemia, and survival to hospital discharge) was higher in studies in which most participants received catheter-directed fibrinolytic therapy compared with those in which patients underwent percutaneous mechanical thrombectomy without local fibrinolysis (91.2 % vs. 82.8 %, p = 0.01) [32]. In general, catheter-assisted techniques combining low-dose "local" fibrinolysis and thrombus fragmentation or aspiration offer the greatest success rate. In a meta-analysis of 35 studies, the overall clinical success rate for catheter-directed therapy was 86.5 % with a relatively low rate of minor (7.9 %) and major (2.4 %) procedural complications [32].

Adjunctive Therapy for Patients with Massive Pulmonary Embolism

Adjunctive therapy for patients with massive PE can be particularly challenging even with the institution of advanced therapy (Table 7.2). While considering advanced therapy, high-dose unfractionated heparin should be administered as soon as massive PE is suspected [7]. The majority of patients will require at least a 10,000-unit bolus of unfractionated heparin followed by a continuous infusion of at least 1250 units/h with a target aPTT of at least 80 s. The rationale for using high doses of heparin is derived from the observation that standard doses often fail to achieve adequate therapeutic anticoagulation, and in patients with massive PE, sub-therapeutic heparin dosing can be fatal.

Although the initial strategy to manage hemodynamic instability is often to augment RV preload with bolus administration of intravenous fluids such as normal saline, care must be taken to avoid excessive volume resuscitation, which may exacerbate RV failure. In the setting of RV pressure overload, volume loading may overdistend the RV, increase wall stress, worsen RV ischemia, decrease contractility, and cause further interventricular septal shift toward the LV, thereby limiting LV filling and reducing systemic cardiac output [33]. An initial trial of 500 ml of normal saline is most likely to be successful in patients without signs of increased right-sided preload, such as those with central venous pressures of less than 12–15 mmHg. In patients with central venous pressures of greater than 12–15 mmHg, volume loading should be avoided, and the administration of vasopressors and inotropes should

Table 7.2 Tips for the supportive care of patients with massive pulmonary embolism (PE)

While considering advanced therapy, high-dose unfractionated heparin should be administered as soon as massive PE is suspected
Higher doses of heparin are often necessary because standard doses frequently fail to achieve adequate therapeutic anticoagulation in patients with massive PE
Care must be taken to avoid excessive volume resuscitation that may worsen right ventricular (RV) failure
An initial trial of modest volume loading such as normal saline 500 ml is most likely to be successful in patients without signs of increased right-sided preload such as those with central venous pressures of less than 12–15 mmHg
In patients with central venous pressures of greater than 12–15 mmHg, volume loading should be avoided and the administration of vasopressors and inotropes should be the first step in hemodynamic support
Norepinephrine, epinephrine, and dopamine are favorable agents for the initial support of patients with massive PE
If an inotrope such as dobutamine is necessary to enhance cardiac output, the addition of a vasopressor may help compensate for inotrope-induced vasodilation and thereby maintain systemic perfusion pressure
In some patients with massive PE and tachycardia, a vasopressor such as vasopressin or phenylephrine may be most appropriate to avoid accelerating the heart rate further
Use vasopressor agents as a "bridge" to more definitive advanced therapy for PE

be the first step in hemodynamic support. In general, vasopressors and inotropes should be administered as a "bridge" to definitive catheter-intervention, surgical intervention, or systemic fibrinolysis.

The ideal agent for the hemodynamic support of patients with massive PE should augment RV function through positive inotropic effects while also maintaining systemic arterial perfusion [33]. Norepinephrine, epinephrine, and dopamine have dual mechanisms of action as both inotropes and vasopressors and therefore may be preferred agents for the initial support of patients with massive PE (Appendix). Inotropes such as dobutamine may be necessary to enhance cardiac output but may also cause systemic arterial hypotension. In such cases, the addition of a vasopressor may be required to maintain systemic perfusion while administering intotropes. In some patients with massive PE and tachycardia, a vasopressor such as vasopressin or phenylephrine may be most appropriate to avoid accelerating the heart rate further.

Extracorporeal Membrane Oxygenation

Extracorporeal membrane oxygenation (ECMO) provides hemodynamic and ventilator support for patients with severe RV failure and cardiogenic shock due to acute PE [34]. Emergency veno-arterial ECMO bypasses the obstructed pulmonary arterial bed, relieving RV pressure overload. In contrast to RV assist devices, veno-arterial ECMO does not further increase pulmonary artery pressures. Utilization of ECMO has been limited by availability and uncertainty about its role for support of patients with acute PE. Until its place in the management of acute PE is defined, ECMO may be considered in PE patients with refractory RV failure and cardiogenic shock.

Pulmonary Embolism Response Teams

Multidisciplinary PE Response Teams merge the expertise of specialists in Cardiovascular Medicine, Pulmonary Medicine, Endovascular Intervention, Cardiac Surgery, and Radiology in order to identify optimal treatment strategies for patients with PE and increased risk for adverse outcomes [35]. PE Response Teams provide rapid evaluation of patients with acute PE and facilitate access to advanced therapies such as systemic fibrinolysis, catheter-directed pharmacomechanical therapy, surgical pulmonary embolectomy, and IVC filter insertion. Such teams are also critical in the utilization of advanced techniques for critically-ill PE patients such as ECMO. A PE Response Team evaluated the patient in the Clinical Vignette, and options for advanced therapy to treat his massive PE were reviewed with the patient, his family, and the Emergency Medicine team. After contraindications to systemic full-dose fibrinolysis were excluded, the patient received the FDA-approved regimen of t-PA 100 mg infused over 2 h. He responded well to fibrinolytic therapy without any bleeding complications.

Answer Key

1. **Correct answer**, (**b**) Large meta-analyses have demonstrated a reduction in all-cause mortality with systemic fibrinolysis in patients with massive or submassive PE. This benefit, however, comes at the price of increased risk of major bleeding, in particular intracranial hemorrhage.
2. **Correct answer**, (**c**) Recent major surgery is a contraindication to any fibrinolytic-based strategy. An IVC filter will prevent subsequent PE but will not reverse the RV failure and hemodynamic deterioration of this patient. Surgical pulmonary embolectomy is an appropriate choice for the patient with massive PE who requires urgent relief of RV pressure overload.

References

1. Kucher N. Clinical practice. Deep-vein thrombosis of the upper extremities. N Engl J Med. 2011;364:861–9.
2. Engelberger RP, Kucher N. Management of deep vein thrombosis of the upper extremity. Circulation. 2012;126:768–73.
3. Russell CE, Wadhera RK, Piazza G. Mesenteric vein thrombosis. Circulation. 2015;131:1599–603.
4. Piazza G. Cerebral venous thrombosis. Circulation. 2012;125:1704–9.
5. Piazza G. Submassive pulmonary embolism. JAMA. 2013;309:171–80.
6. Karthikesalingam A, Young EL, Hinchliffe RJ, Loftus IM, Thompson MM, Holt PJ. A systematic review of percutaneous mechanical thrombectomy in the treatment of deep venous thrombosis. Eur J Vasc Endovasc Surg. 2011;41:554–65.
7. Piazza G, Goldhaber SZ. Fibrinolysis for acute pulmonary embolism. Vasc Med. 2010;15:419–28.
8. Becattini C, Agnelli G, Salvi A, et al. Bolus tenecteplase for right ventricle dysfunction in hemodynamically stable patients with pulmonary embolism. Thromb Res. 2010;125:e82–6.
9. Goldhaber SZ, Come PC, Lee RT, et al. Alteplase versus heparin in acute pulmonary embolism: randomised trial assessing right-ventricular function and pulmonary perfusion. Lancet. 1993;341:507–11.
10. Nass N, McConnell MV, Goldhaber SZ, Chyu S, Solomon SD. Recovery of regional right ventricular function after thrombolysis for pulmonary embolism. Am J Cardiol. 1999;83:804–6.
11. Sharma GV, Burleson VA, Sasahara AA. Effect of thrombolytic therapy on pulmonary-capillary blood volume in patients with pulmonary embolism. N Engl J Med. 1980;303:842–5.
12. Kline JA, Steuerwald MT, Marchick MR, Hernandez-Nino J, Rose GA. Prospective evaluation of right ventricular function and functional status 6 months after acute submassive pulmonary embolism: frequency of persistent or subsequent elevation in estimated pulmonary artery pressure. Chest. 2009;136:1202–10.
13. Sharifi M, Bay C, Skrocki L, Rahimi F, Mehdipour M, Investigators M. Moderate pulmonary embolism treated with thrombolysis (from the "MOPETT" Trial). Am J Cardiol. 2013;111:273–7.
14. Sharma GV, Folland ED, McIntyre KM, Sasahara AA. Long-term benefit of thrombolytic therapy in patients with pulmonary embolism. Vasc Med. 2000;5:91–5.
15. Jaff MR, McMurtry MS, Archer SL, et al. Management of massive and submassive pulmonary embolism, iliofemoral deep vein thrombosis, and chronic thromboembolic pulmonary hypertension: a scientific statement from the American Heart Association. Circulation. 2011;123:1788–830.

16. Kearon C, Akl EA, Comerota AJ, et al. Antithrombotic therapy for VTE disease: antithrombotic therapy and prevention of thrombosis, 9th ed: American College of Chest Physicians Evidence-Based Clinical Practice Guidelines. Chest. 2012;141:e419S–94.
17. Konstantinides SV, Torbicki A, Agnelli G, et al. 2014 ESC Guidelines on the diagnosis and management of acute pulmonary embolism: the Task Force for the Diagnosis and Management of Acute Pulmonary Embolism of the European Society of Cardiology (ESC) Endorsed by the European Respiratory Society (ERS). Eur Heart J. 2014;35:3033–73.
18. Meyer G, Vicaut E, Danays T, et al. Fibrinolysis for patients with intermediate-risk pulmonary embolism. N Engl J Med. 2014;370:1402–11.
19. Chatterjee S, Chakraborty A, Weinberg I, et al. Thrombolysis for pulmonary embolism and risk of all-cause mortality, major bleeding, and intracranial hemorrhage: a meta-analysis. JAMA. 2014;311:2414–21.
20. Marti C, John G, Konstantinides S, et al. Systemic thrombolytic therapy for acute pulmonary embolism: a systematic review and meta-analysis. Eur Heart J. 2015;36:605–14.
21. Fiumara K, Kucher N, Fanikos J, Goldhaber SZ. Predictors of major hemorrhage following fibrinolysis for acute pulmonary embolism. Am J Cardiol. 2006;97:127–9.
22. Goldhaber SZ, Visani L, De Rosa M. Acute pulmonary embolism: clinical outcomes in the International Cooperative Pulmonary Embolism Registry (ICOPER). Lancet. 1999;353: 1386–9.
23. Wang C, Zhai Z, Yang Y, et al. Efficacy and safety of low dose recombinant tissue-type plasminogen activator for the treatment of acute pulmonary thromboembolism: a randomized, multicenter, controlled trial. Chest. 2010;137:254–62.
24. Daniels LB, Parker JA, Patel SR, Grodstein F, Goldhaber SZ. Relation of duration of symptoms with response to thrombolytic therapy in pulmonary embolism. Am J Cardiol. 1997;80:184–8.
25. Meneveau N, Bassand JP, Schiele F, et al. Safety of thrombolytic therapy in elderly patients with massive pulmonary embolism: a comparison with nonelderly patients. J Am Coll Cardiol. 1993;22:1075–9.
26. Aklog L, Williams CS, Byrne JG, Goldhaber SZ. Acute pulmonary embolectomy: a contemporary approach. Circulation. 2002;105:1416–9.
27. Leacche M, Unic D, Goldhaber SZ, et al. Modern surgical treatment of massive pulmonary embolism: results in 47 consecutive patients after rapid diagnosis and aggressive surgical approach. J Thorac Cardiovasc Surg. 2005;129:1018–23.
28. Enden T, Haig Y, Klow NE, et al. Long-term outcome after additional catheter-directed thrombolysis versus standard treatment for acute iliofemoral deep vein thrombosis (the CaVenT study): a randomised controlled trial. Lancet. 2012;379:31–8.
29. Kucher N. Catheter embolectomy for acute pulmonary embolism. Chest. 2007;132:657–63.
30. Kucher N, Boekstegers P, Muller O, et al. Randomized controlled trial of ultrasound-assisted catheter-directed thrombolysis for acute intermediate-risk pulmonary embolism. Circulation. 2014;129:479–86.
31. Piazza G, Hohlfelder B, Jaff MR, et al. A prospective, single-arm, multicenter trial of ultrasound-facilitated catheter-directed low-dose fibrinolysis for acute massive and submassive pulmonary embolism (SEATTLE II). JACC Cardiovasc Interv. 2015; in press.
32. Kuo WT, Gould MK, Louie JD, Rosenberg JK, Sze DY, Hofmann LV. Catheter-directed therapy for the treatment of massive pulmonary embolism: systematic review and meta-analysis of modern techniques. J Vasc Interv Radiol. 2009;20:1431–40.
33. Piazza G, Goldhaber SZ. The acutely decompensated right ventricle: pathways for diagnosis and management. Chest. 2005;128:1836–52.
34. Belohlavek J, Rohn V, Jansa P, et al. Veno-arterial ECMO in severe acute right ventricular failure with pulmonary obstructive hemodynamic pattern. J Invasive Cardiol. 2010;22: 365–9.
35. Kabrhel C, Jaff MR, Channick RN, Baker JN, Rosenfield K. A multidisciplinary pulmonary embolism response team. Chest. 2013;144:1738–9.

Chapter 8
Inferior Vena Cava Filters: Recognizing Indications for Placement and Retrieval

Abstract Inferior vena cava (IVC) filter placement is indicated in patients with acute pulmonary embolism (PE) or deep vein thrombosis (PE) who have contraindications to anticoagulation or who have recurrent PE despite therapeutic anticoagulation. IVC filter insertion may be considered on a case-by-case basis for patients with acute PE who are able to receive therapeutic anticoagulation but who have limited cardiopulmonary reserve and in whom a subsequent PE would likely be fatal. Retrievable IVC filters are inserted to provide temporary protection from PE during such periods of increased vulnerability or when interruption of anticoagulation is necessary. IVC filters should be retrieved as soon as they are no longer necessary.

Keywords Deep vein thrombosis • Inferior vena cava filter • Pulmonary embolism • Venous thromboembolism

Self-Assessment Questions

1. Which of the following statements regarding IVC filters for treatment of patients with acute PE is false?

   (a) IVC filters are indicated for patients with contraindications to anticoagulation or with recurrent PE despite therapeutic anticoagulation.
   (b) IVC filters decrease the risk of PE in the short-term but increase the long-term risk of deep vein thrombosis (DVT).
   (c) Retrievable IVC filters should be left in place permanently even if a transient contraindication to anticoagulation has resolved.
   (d) IVC filters have little impact on the in-hospital mortality rate of hemodynamically stable patients with acute PE.

2. In which of the following patients is IVC filter retrieval appropriate?

   (a) A 92-year-old woman with history of massive PE and recurrent severe upper gastrointestinal bleeding episodes due to gastric antral vascular ectasia.
   (b) A 24-year-old man with extensive left lower extremity DVT and bilateral PE following a motor vehicle accident with multiple fractures who was restarted on therapeutic anticoagulation 3 months ago and has been stable.

(c) A 69-year-old man with early stage colon cancer status resection compli-
    cated by post-operative bilateral PE who is planned for ostomy reversal in 3
    months.
(d) An 82-year-old woman with cerebral amyloid angiopathy complicated by
    intracranial hemorrhage while on therapeutic anticoagulation for unpro-
    voked bilateral PE.

Clinical Vignette
A 44-year-old morbidly obese man with ventral hernia repair 3 weeks prior
presented to the Emergency Department with 48 h of progressive dyspnea
at rest and with exertion. One week prior to presentation, the patient noted
right calf cramping with ambulation. He attributed this to being relatively
sedentary since his surgery. On physical examination, he was tachycardic
to 130 beats per minute, hypotensive with a blood pressure of 82/44 mmHg,
and hypoxemic with an oxygen saturation of 88 % on room air. His electrocardiogram was notable for sinus tachycardia to the 130 s. His chest
X-ray demonstrated a small left pleural effusion. Contrast-enhanced chest
computed tomogram (CT) demonstrated a large bilateral PE and right ventricular (RV) enlargement with an RV diameter-to-left ventricular (LV)
diameter ratio of 1.4. In the Emergency Department, the patient's blood
pressure increased to 100/68 mmHg following a 1 L normal saline bolus.
He was started on intravenous unfractionated heparin as a bolus and then
continuous infusion with a target activated partial thromboplastin time
(aPTT) of 60–80 s. Right lower extremity venous ultrasound demonstrated
common femoral, femoral, popliteal, gastrocnemius, peroneal, and posterior tibial DVT. Because of the large reservoir of thrombus in the patient's
right lower extremity and the concern that a subsequent PE might be fatal,
the Emergency Department physician consulted the hospital's multidisciplinary PE Response Team. The PE Response Team determined that a fibrinolytic based approach was contraindicated given his recent surgery and
that his morbid obesity increased the operative risk of surgical pulmonary
embolectomy. Therefore, the PE Response Team arranged for a retrievable IVC filter to be placed in the Cardiac Catheterization Laboratory
(Fig. 8.1). After insertion of the IVC filter, the patient was admitted to the
Intensive Care Unit and then transferred to a floor bed the following day.
He remained hemodynamically stable, and his dyspnea and hypoxemia
resolved on therapeutic anticoagulation. He was subsequently discharged
on oral anticoagulation with warfarin and arranged to follow-up in Vascular
Medicine clinic. Six weeks after hospital discharge, he had fully recov-
ered, and his Vascular Medicine physician arranged for IVC filter retrieval
(Figs. 8.2, 8.3, and 8.4).

Fig. 8.1 Successful insertion of a retrievable inferior vena cava (IVC) filter (*arrow*) under fluoroscopy in a 44-year-old morbidly obese man with a ventral hernia repair 3 weeks prior who presented with severe dyspnea and was diagnosed with massive pulmonary embolism (PE) and extensive right lower extremity deep vein thrombosis (DVT)

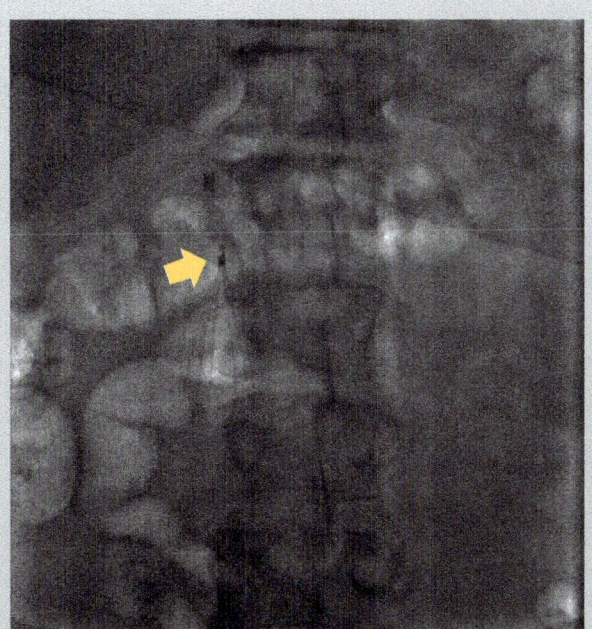

Fig. 8.2 Fluoroscopy demonstrating a well-positioned intact retrievable inferior vena cava (IVC) filter 6 weeks after insertion in a 44-year-old morbidly obese man with a massive pulmonary embolism (PE) and extensive right lower extremity deep vein thrombosis (DVT). The retrieval hook (*arrow*) is easily accessible from a superior approach

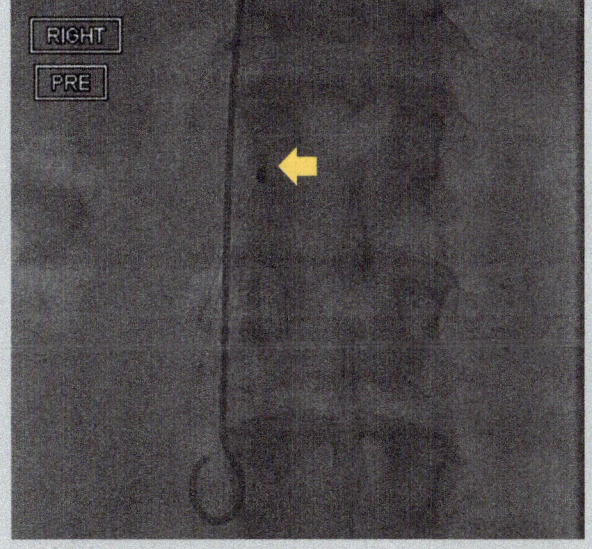

Fig. 8.3 Contrast cavogram demonstrating a patent inferior vena cava (IVC) and a retrievable IVC filter that is free of thrombus 6 weeks after insertion in a 44-year-old morbidly obese man with a massive pulmonary embolism (PE) and extensive right lower extremity deep vein thrombosis (DVT)

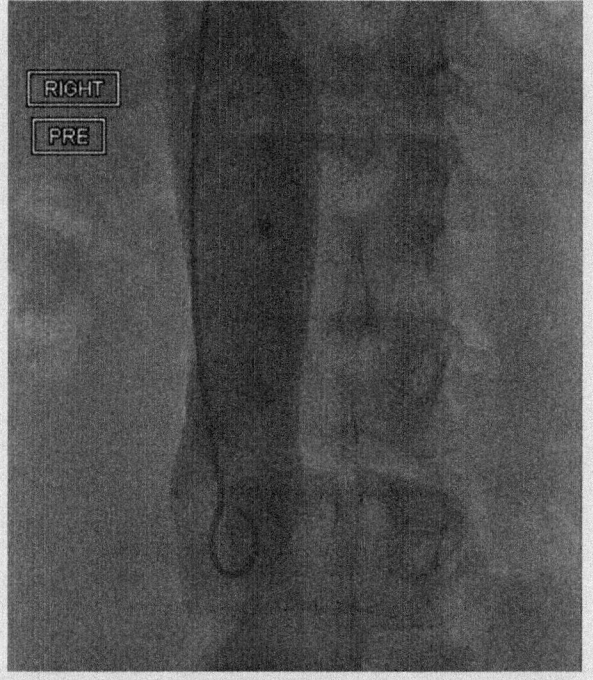

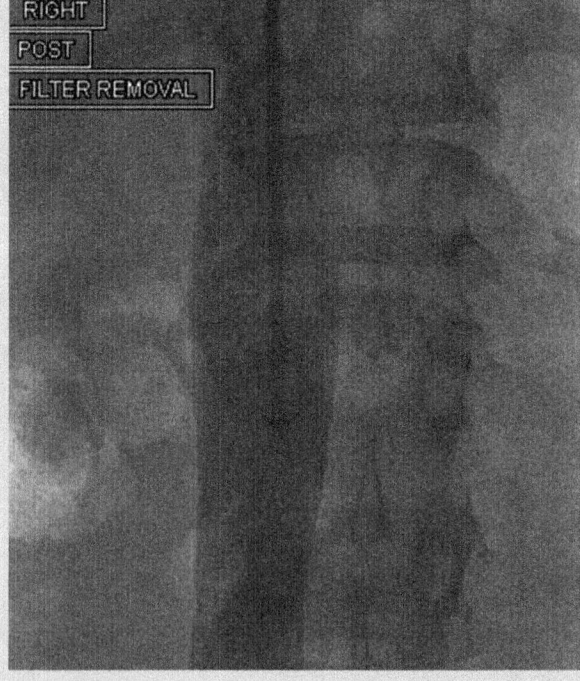

Fig. 8.4 Completion contrast cavogram following inferior vena cava (IVC) filter retrieval 6 weeks after insertion in a 44-year-old morbidly obese man with a massive pulmonary embolism (PE) and extensive right lower extremity deep vein thrombosis (DVT). The IVC filter has been completed retrieved, and the IVC appears intact without thrombus

An analysis of data from the National Hospital Discharge Survey spanning 1979–2006 demonstrated that utilization of both permanent and retrievable IVC filters has increased in the U.S. [1]. IVC filter insertion increased threefold from 2001 through 2006. A retrospective community-based study demonstrated that IVC filter insertion was deemed appropriate in only half of cases [2].

Indications

IVC filter insertion should be considered in patients with objectively-confirmed acute PE or DVT and contraindications to anticoagulation or with recurrent PE despite therapeutic anticoagulation (Table 8.1) [3–5]. Insertion of an IVC filter may be considered on an individual basis for patients with acute PE who are able to receive therapeutic anticoagulation but who have limited cardiopulmonary reserve, such that a subsequent PE would likely be fatal. The patient in the Clinical Vignette provides an example of a patient with acute PE who was able to receive therapeutic anticoagulation but was not eligible for any advanced therapies and in whom a subsequent PE would have been potentially fatal. An IVC filter was inserted in this patient until he had survived the acute vulnerable period.

IVC filter insertion may also be considered in patients with high risk of PE in the setting of major surgery or trauma and who are unable to receive even prophylactic-level anticoagulation for a prolonged period of time. Although data regarding their use in these setting are limited, IVC filters are frequently inserted in patients undergoing surgical pulmonary embolectomy for acute PE, pulmonary thromboendarterectomy for chronic thromboembolic pulmonary hypertension, and catheter-directed therapy for iliofemoral or femoral DVT.

Retrievable IVC filters offer a safe and effective alternative to permanent filters and may be removed up to several months after insertion in patients with transient contraindications to anticoagulation [6].

Table 8.1 Major indications for inferior vena cava (IVC) filter insertion

Objectively-confirmed acute pulmonary embolism (PE) or deep vein thrombosis (DVT) and contraindications to anticoagulation
Recurrent PE despite therapeutic anticoagulation
Patients with acute PE who are anticoagulated but who have limited cardiopulmonary reserve, such that a subsequent PE may be fatal
Patients with high risk of PE in the setting of major surgery or trauma and who are unable to receive even prophylactic-level anticoagulation for a prolonged period of time
Patients undergoing surgical pulmonary embolectomy for acute PE
Patients undergoing pulmonary thromboendarterectomy for chronic thromboembolic pulmonary hypertension
Patients undergoing catheter-directed therapy for iliofemoral or femoral DVT

Understanding the Evidence

While they reduce the short-term risk of PE in patients with acute VTE [7], IVC filters neither halt the thrombotic process nor treat acute pulmonary hypertension and RV pressure overload. An analysis of the Healthcare Cost and Utilization Project (HCUP) Nationwide Inpatient Sample demonstrated that the in-hospital case fatality rate was only marginally lower in stable patients with acute PE who received IVC filters than in those who did not (7.2 % vs. 7.9 %, $p < 0.0001$) [8]. However, unstable patients with acute PE who received IVC filters had substantial reductions in in-hospital case fatality rate compared with those who did not, whether (7.6 % vs. 18 %, $p < 0.0001$) or not (33 % vs. 51 %, $p < 0.0001$) fibrinolytic therapy was administered. An analysis of the International Cooperative Pulmonary Embolism Registry (ICOPER) noted a significant reduction in 90-day mortality associated with the use of IVC filters [9].

Limitations

Permanent IVC filters increase the long-term risk of DVT [7]. Despite data demonstrating the safety and ease with which retrievable IVC filters can be removed, a number of studies have shown that a substantial proportion of retrievable IVC filters are left permanently indwelling [10, 11]. Reported IVC filter retrieval rates have ranged from less than 10 to 50 % [10, 11]. Retrieval rates of IVC filters appear to be most influenced by insurance status, distance from the medical center, and age [12]. Quality Improvement initiatives are effective in increasing IVC filter retrieval rates. In one study, rates of IVC filter insertion increased from 8 to 40 % with the mailing of clinician reminder letters and to 52 % with the automated scheduling of a clinic visit 4 weeks after IVC filter placement [11].

Increasing utilization of retrievable IVC filters has raised awareness of device-associated complications. Device-related complications appear to occur with significantly higher frequency with retrievable IVC filters than permanent models [13]. Reported device-related complications include strut fracture, filter migration, strut embolization, device tilt, IVC penetration, perforation of surrounding structures, including the aorta and small intestine, PE, DVT, IVC thrombus, and malfunction during placement (Table 8.2 and Fig. 8.5).

Practical Considerations

In the vast majority of cases, a retrievable IVC filter should be selected instead of a permanent model (Table 8.3). Patients and primary providers should be advised that the goal of the IVC filter is to provide temporary protection from PE and that the device will be retrieved as soon as it is no longer necessary (Fig. 8.6). Providers should schedule a follow-up visit with a specialist who can decide if and when the

Table 8.2 Complications of inferior vena cava (IVC) filters

IVC filter migration
Strut fracture
Strut embolization
Device tilt
IVC penetration
Perforation of surrounding structures, including the aorta and small intestine
Pulmonary embolism
Deep vein thrombosis
IVC thrombus
Malfunction during placement

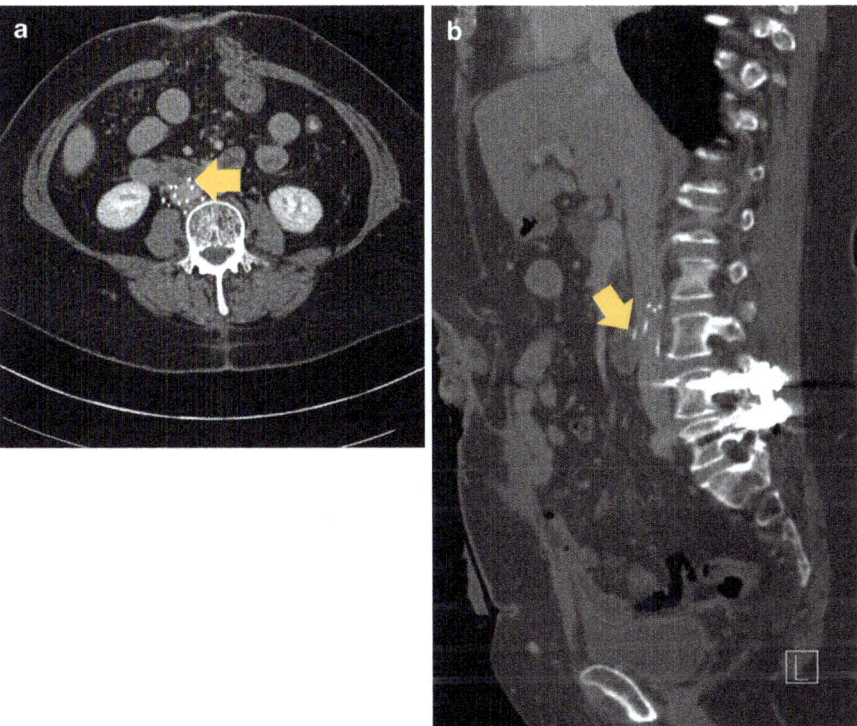

Fig. 8.5 Contrast-enhanced abdominal computed tomogram (CT) demonstrating several inferior vena cava (IVC) filter struts protruding through the wall of the IVC in a 54-year-old woman with history of recurrent pulmonary embolism who presented with several weeks of abdominal and back pain (**panels a** and **b**). One strut has perforated the duodenum (*arrows*)

IVC filter should be retrieved. The patient in the Clinical Vignette was provided follow-up in Vascular Medicine clinic. The Vascular Medicine physician determined that the IVC filter was no longer needed and arranged for it to be retrieved. Many Medical Centers have instituted effective "reminder" systems, either by email or by

Table 8.3 Practical considerations for inferior vena cava (IVC) filter insertion

In the majority of cases, a retrievable IVC filter should be selected instead of a permanent model
Patients and primary providers should be advised that the goal of the IVC filter is to provide temporary protection from pulmonary embolism (PE) and that the device will be retrieved as soon as it is no longer necessary
Providers should schedule a follow-up visit with a specialist who can decide if and when the IVC filter should be retrieved
Interventionalists placing retrievable IVC filters should be cognizant of the recommended retrieval interval for a particular model
IVC filters should be avoided in patients with suspected or documented heparin-induced thrombocytopenia (HIT) and advanced malignancy because of the risk of caval thrombosis
Suprarenal placement of IVC filters is associated with increased risk of complications such as device migration and malalignment
Anticoagulation should be started in all VTE patients with an IVC filter as soon as the transient contraindication to anticoagulant therapy is no longer present

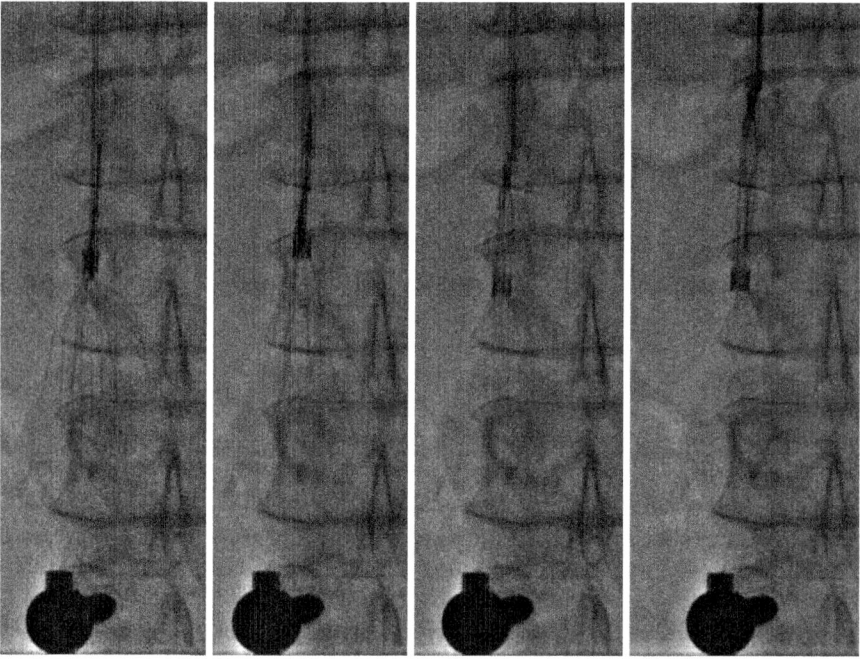

Fig. 8.6 Fluoroscopic retrieval of an inferior vena cava (IVC) filter, via right internal jugular vein approach, in a 54-year-old woman with history of recurrent pulmonary embolism who presented a device strut perforating the duodenum. The IVC filter retrieval hook is engaged and partially withdrawn into the retrieval sheath (leftward-most panel). The IVC filter is then gradually withdrawn until it is completely collapsed within the retrieval sheath (subsequent panels). The IVC filter and retrieval sheath are then removed from the patient

letter, to notify providers that IVC filters should be retrieved when no longer needed. Interventionalists placing retrievable IVC filters should be cognizant of the recommended retrieval interval for a particular model. In general, retrievable IVC filters can be successfully removed up to several months after insertion. Advanced techniques, including snare retrieval and laser sheath excision, have been used by experienced operators to remove filters that have failed usual retrieval methods or ones that have been in place for a protracted length of time [14].

IVC filters should be avoided, if possible, in certain patient populations because of the risk of thromboembolic complications. IVC filters in patients with suspected or documented heparin-induced thrombocytopenia (HIT) have been associated with devastating caval thrombosis. Likewise, IVC filters should be avoided in patients with advanced cancer because the prothrombotic state of malignancy can increase the risk of IVC filter thrombosis. In contrast to placement below the renal veins (infrarenal), suprarenal IVC filters are associated with increased risk of complications such as device migration and malalignment. Superior vena cava (SVC) filters should also be avoided because of the increased risk of SVC syndrome should the filter become occluded.

Anticoagulation should be started in all VTE patients with an IVC filter as soon as the transient contraindication to anticoagulant therapy is no longer present. A common clinical question is whether a chronically indwelling IVC filter is an indication for indefinite duration anticoagulation regardless of the patient's risk for recurrent VTE. Given a paucity of clinical trial data, clinical practice guidelines suggest that the decision regarding duration of anticoagulation in patients with indwelling IVC filters be made primarily on the basis of risk of VTE recurrence [15].

Answer Key

1. **Correct answer**, (**c**) Once a transient contraindication to anticoagulation has resolved, anticoagulant therapy should be initiated and plans for IVC filter retrieval should be made in order to avoid long-term filter-related complications such as device fragmentation or migration and IVC thrombosis.
2. **Correct answer**, (**b**) The 24-year-old man with extensive left lower extremity DVT and bilateral PE following a motor vehicle accident has tolerated therapeutic anticoagulation without bleeding and is a candidate for IVC filter retrieval. Each of the other patients has an ongoing indication for an IVC filter due to the inability to be safely anticoagulated or the need for further anticoagulation interruption for a procedure.

References

1. Stein PD, Matta F, Hull RD. Increasing use of vena cava filters for prevention of pulmonary embolism. Am J Med. 2011;124:655–61.
2. Spencer FA, Bates SM, Goldberg RJ, et al. A population-based study of inferior vena cava filters in patients with acute venous thromboembolism. Arch Intern Med. 2010;170:1456–62.

 3. Jaff MR, McMurtry MS, Archer SL, et al. Management of massive and submassive pulmonary embolism, iliofemoral deep vein thrombosis, and chronic thromboembolic pulmonary hypertension: a scientific statement from the American Heart Association. Circulation. 2011;123: 1788–830.
 4. Kearon C, Akl EA, Comerota AJ, et al. Antithrombotic therapy for VTE disease: antithrombotic therapy and prevention of thrombosis, 9th ed: American College of Chest Physicians Evidence-Based Clinical Practice Guidelines. Chest. 2012;141:e419S–94.
 5. Konstantinides SV, Torbicki A, Agnelli G, et al. 2014 ESC Guidelines on the diagnosis and management of acute pulmonary embolism: the Task Force for the Diagnosis and Management of Acute Pulmonary Embolism of the European Society of Cardiology (ESC) Endorsed by the European Respiratory Society (ERS). Eur Heart J. 2014;35:3033–73.
 6. Mismetti P, Rivron-Guillot K, Quenet S, et al. A prospective long-term study of 220 patients with a retrievable vena cava filter for secondary prevention of venous thromboembolism. Chest. 2007;131:223–9.
 7. Decousus H, Leizorovicz A, Parent F, et al. A clinical trial of vena caval filters in the prevention of pulmonary embolism in patients with proximal deep-vein thrombosis. Prevention du Risque d'Embolie Pulmonaire par Interruption Cave Study Group. N Engl J Med. 1998;338: 409–15.
 8. Stein PD, Matta F, Keyes DC, Willyerd GL. Impact of vena cava filters on in-hospital case fatality rate from pulmonary embolism. Am J Med. 2012;125:478–84.
 9. Kucher N, Rossi E, De Rosa M, Goldhaber SZ. Massive pulmonary embolism. Circulation. 2006;113:577–82.
10. Rottenstreich A, Spectre G, Roth B, Bloom AI, Kalish Y. Patterns of use and outcome of inferior vena cava filters in a tertiary care setting. Eur J Haematol. 2015 Mar 6. [Epub ahead of print].
11. Sutphin PD, Reis SP, McKune A, Ravanzo M, Kalva SP, Pillai AK. Improving inferior vena cava filter retrieval rates with the define, measure, analyze, improve, control methodology. J Vasc Interv Radiol. 2015;26:491–8.
12. Smith SC, Shanks C, Guy G, Yang X, Dowell JD. Social and demographic factors influencing inferior vena cava filter retrieval at a single institution in the United States. Cardiovasc Intervent Radiol. 2014 Dec 31. [Epub ahead of print].
13. Andreoli JM, Lewandowski RJ, Vogelzang RL, Ryu RK. Comparison of complication rates associated with permanent and retrievable inferior vena cava filters: a review of the MAUDE database. J Vasc Interv Radiol. 2014;25:1181–5.
14. Kuo WT, Cupp JS, Louie JD, et al. Complex retrieval of embedded IVC filters: alternative techniques and histologic tissue analysis. Cardiovasc Intervent Radiol. 2012;35:588–97.
15. British Committee for Standards in Haematology, Writing G, Baglin TP, Brush J, Streiff M. Guidelines on use of vena cava filters. Br J Haematol. 2006;134:590–5.

Chapter 9
Anticoagulation for Venous Thromboembolism: Selecting the Optimal Parenteral and Oral Anticoagulant Regimen

Abstract Prompt therapeutic-level anticoagulation is the cornerstone of treatment for venous thromboembolism (VTE). Options for anticoagulation in VTE include unfractionated heparin, low-molecular-weight heparin, fondaparinux, argatroban, bivalirudin, warfarin, and the non-vitamin K oral anticoagulants (NOACs) rivaroxaban, dabigatran, apixaban, and edoxaban. The NOACs represent a major advance in anticoagulation for VTE with superior safety and equivalent efficacy compared with warfarin.

Keywords Anticoagulation • Heparin • Low-molecular weight heparin • NOACs • Non-vitamin K oral anticoagulants • Warfarin

Self-Assessment Questions

1. Which of the following anticoagulation regimens for VTE treatment is correct?

    (a) Dalteparin 200 units/kg subcutaneously once daily in a patient with advanced breast cancer and acute pulmonary embolism (PE).
    (b) Dabigatran 150 mg orally twice daily in a patient with subclavian vein thrombosis associated with a hemodialysis access catheter.
    (c) Warfarin with a target International Normalized Ratio (INR) range of 2–3 in a patient receiving total parenteral nutrition (TPN) for chronic pancreatitis and malabsorption and suffered lower extremity deep vein thrombosis (DVT).
    (d) Enoxaparin 1 mg/kg subcutaneously twice daily in a patient with a remote history of heparin-induced thrombocytopenia who presents with acute PE.

2. Which of the following statements about use of NOACs for treatment of VTE is correct?

    (a) NOACs are comparable to warfarin with regard to cost burden to the patient.
    (b) NOACs have been proven to be non-inferior with regard to efficacy and superior with regard to bleeding complications compared with warfarin.
    (c) NOACs are preferred in patients who have difficulty remembering to take their medications as directed.
    (d) Apixaban and edoxaban are administered as completely oral monotherapy with a loading dose followed by a maintenance dose.

© Springer International Publishing Switzerland 2015   77
G. Piazza et al., *Handbook for Venous Thromboembolism*,
DOI 10.1007/978-3-319-20843-5_9

3. Which of the following strategies for treating anticoagulant-associated major bleeding is not correct?

(a) Protamine for intravenous unfractionated heparin
(b) Prothrombin complex concentrate for warfarin
(c) Hemodialysis for apixaban overdose
(d) Prothrombin complex concentrate for rivaroxaban

Clinical Vignette

A 54-year-old man presented to the Emergency Department 3 weeks following L4-L5 laminectomy and fusion with acute dyspnea and right-sided pleuritic flank pain. He noted that his mobility had been limited by post-operative pain in the few weeks since hospital discharge. On physical examination, he had a heart rate of 82 beats per minute, a blood pressure of 126/78 mmHg, and an oxygen saturation of 92 % on room air. Because of his post-operative state and a high suspicion for PE, the patient proceeded directly to contrast-enhanced chest computed tomogram (CT). The study demonstrated a right lower lobe subsegmental PE (Fig. 9.1) and associated wedge-shaped pleural based opacity consistent with a pulmonary infarct (Fig. 9.2). His chest CT-determined RV diameter-to-LV diameter ratio was normal at 0.89 (Fig. 9.3). The patient was promptly administered intravenous (IV) unfractionated heparin as a bolus followed by infusion titrated to a goal activated partial thromboplastin time (aPTT) of 50–70 s and admitted to the Medical Service. His symptoms and hypoxemia improved over the subsequent 48 h. The Medical Team discussed options for oral anticoagulation with the patient who preferred an agent that did not require routine laboratory monitoring or dose adjustment. The team discharged the patient on one of the non-vitamin K oral anticoagulants.

Regardless of whether patients receive advanced therapy, prompt therapeutic-level anticoagulation remains the cornerstone of treatment for VTE. Currently, U.S. Food and Drug Administration-approved agents for anticoagulation in VTE include unfractionated heparin, low-molecular-weight heparin, fondaparinux, argatroban, bivalirudin, warfarin, and the non-vitamin K oral anticoagulants (NOACs) rivaroxaban, dabigatran, apixaban, and edoxaban. The NOACs, also known as target-specific oral anticoagulants (TSOACs) or direct oral anticoagulants (DOACs), represent a major advancement in anticoagulation for VTE with strong safety and efficacy performance in their respective randomized controlled trials [1–6].

Fig. 9.1 Contrast-enhanced chest computed tomogram (CT) demonstrating right lower lobe subsegmental pulmonary embolism (PE) (*arrow*) in a 54-year-old man with dyspnea and right-sided pleuritic flank pain following spine surgery

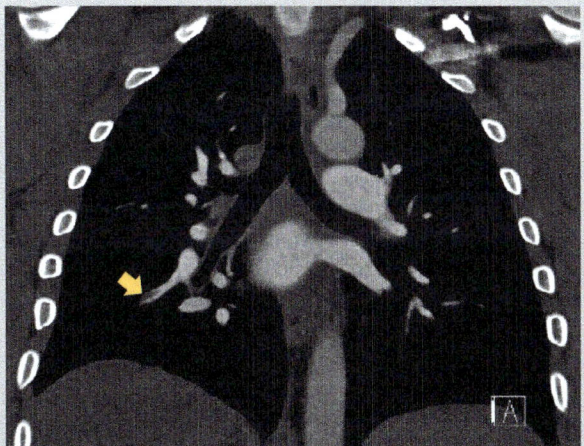

Fig. 9.2 Contrast-enhanced chest computed tomogram (CT) demonstrating a right lower lobe pulmonary infarct (*arrow*) in a 54-year-old man with dyspnea and right-sided pleuritic flank pain and acute pulmonary embolism (PE) following spine surgery

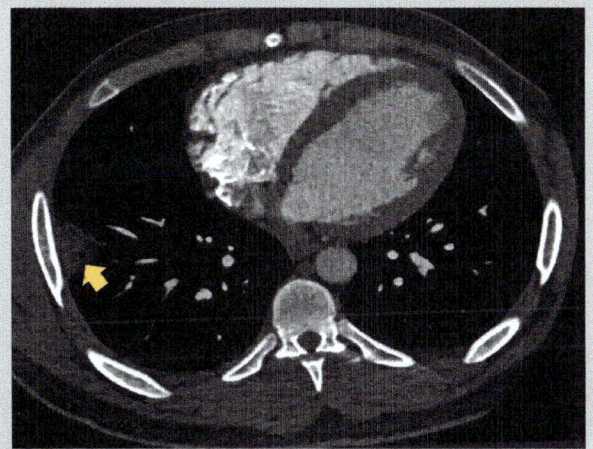

Fig. 9.3 Contrast-enhanced chest computed tomogram (CT) demonstrating normal right ventricular (RV) size as defined by a normal RV diameter-to-left ventricular (LV) diameter ratio (5 cm/5.6 cm = 0.89; normal ≤ 0.9) in a 54-year-old man with acute pulmonary embolism (PE) following spine surgery

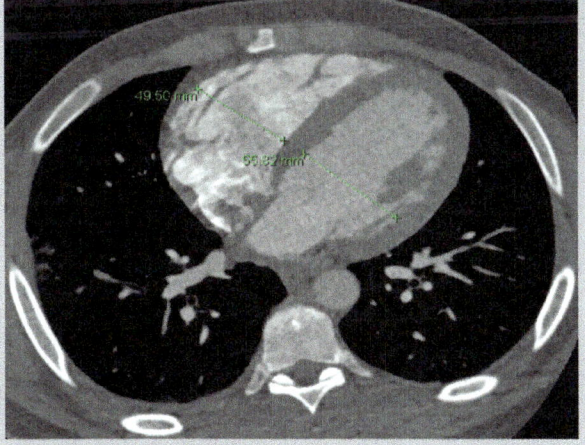

Parenteral Anticoagulation

Unfractionated Heparin

The majority of patients with massive or submassive VTE will initially receive unfractionated heparin administered as an IV bolus, followed by continuous infusion titrated to a goal aPTT of 2–3 times the upper limit of normal, or approximately 60–80 s. Weight-based protocols such as the modified Raschke nomogram are widely used and may more rapidly achieve therapeutic levels of anticoagulation (Table 9.1) [7, 8]. Because it can be discontinued and rapidly reversed, unfractionated heparin is the preferred anticoagulant for patients undergoing advanced therapy with fibrinolysis, catheter-based intervention, or surgery for VTE. Although unfractionated heparin is continued during fibrinolysis for acute myocardial infarction, it is withheld during the administration of systemic dose recombinant tissue-plasminogen activator (t-PA) for VTE and is not restarted until the aPTT has fallen to less than 80 s or twice the upper limit of normal [9]. The patient in the Clinical Vignette was initiated on IV unfractionated heparin as soon as the diagnosis of PE was established.

Low-Molecular Weight Heparin

Low-molecular-weight heparins (LMWHs), including enoxaparin, dalteparin, and tinzaparin, offer several advantages over unfractionated heparin, including longer half-life, more consistent bioavailability, and more predictable dose response. LMWHs are dosed according to weight, administered subcutaneously, and do not require dose adjustments or laboratory monitoring under routine circumstances.

Several trials have demonstrated that LMWHs are at least as safe and effective as IV unfractionated heparin in the prevention of recurrent VTE after DVT [10–12]. A meta-analysis of randomized, controlled trials comparing LMWH therapy with IV unfractionated heparin for the treatment of DVT demonstrated a 30 % reduction in mortality and 40 % reduction in risk of major bleeding associated with LMWH use [11].

Table 9.1 A generally-accepted weight-based unfractionated heparin nomogram

Variable	Heparin dose
Initial heparin dose	80 U/kg bolus, then 18 U/kg/h
aPTT <35 s (<1.2×control)	80 U/kg bolus, then increase infusion by 4 U/kg/h
aPTT 35–59 s (1.2–1.9×control)	40 U/kg bolus, then increase infusion by 2 U/kg/h
aPTT 60–89 s (2.0–2.9×control)	No change
aPTT 90–100 s (3.0–3.3×control)	Decrease infusion by 3 U/kg/h
aPTT >100 s (>3.3×control)	Hold infusion 1 h; then decrease infusion rate by 4 U/kg/h

aPTT activated partial thromboplastin time

The U.S. Food and Drug Administration (FDA) has approved enoxaparin and tinzaparin for treatment of DVT as "bridge" to therapeutic oral anticoagulation. LMWHs have also been shown to be as safe and effective as IV unfractionated heparin in the prevention of recurrent VTE among patients with acute PE [13, 14].

For patients with active cancer, LMWH monotherapy without transition to oral anticoagulation is preferred over warfarin in evidence-based guideline recommendations [15, 16]. In a randomized controlled trial of 676 cancer patients, LMWH monotherapy with dalteparin halved VTE recurrence compared with warfarin (hazard ratio [HR], 0.48; p = 0.002) [17].

In contrast to unfractionated heparin, which is largely eliminated by the liver, LMWHs are cleared renally. Patients with impaired renal clearance, massive obesity, pregnancy, or unanticipated bleeding or thromboembolism despite correct weight-based dosing of LMWH may benefit from laboratory monitoring. Although the aPTT is checked to monitor the level of anticoagulation with unfractionated heparin therapy, anti-Xa levels (often called "heparin levels") are used to determine the level of anticoagulation with LMWHs. The goal therapeutic range for anti-Xa levels is 0.5–1.0 anti-Xa IU/mL. Anti-Xa levels should be drawn 4–6 h after the second or third dose of LMWH to ensure a steady-state value. The use of anti-Xa testing has been the subject of considerable debate because the correlation of anti-Xa levels to antithrombotic effect and risk of bleeding has come into question [18, 19].

Adverse Effects of Heparin

Bleeding is the most common clinically important adverse effect of heparin therapy. Although in most cases discontinuation of heparin therapy is sufficient, protamine sulfate may be necessary to reverse the effects of heparin in the setting of life-threatening hemorrhage. Protamine sulfate is administered as a slow IV infusion in a dose of 1 mg for every 100 units of heparin administered over the preceding 4 h, up to a maximum dose of 50 mg. A potentially severe allergic reaction may occur in patients who have been exposed to Neutral Protamine Hagedorn (NPH) insulin. In general, major bleeding from the respiratory, gastrointestinal, or genitourinary tracts should not be attributed to anticoagulation alone, and an evaluation for a source of bleeding such as malignancy should be undertaken after the acute illness has resolved.

Other important potential adverse effects of heparin therapy include heparin-induced bone loss and thrombocytopenia.

Heparin-Induced Thrombocytopenia

Heparin-induced thrombocytopenia (HIT) is caused by heparin-dependent IgG antibodies directed against heparin-platelet factor 4 complex. Although bleeding is a rare complication of HIT, devastating arterial and, more commonly, venous thromboembolic complications may culminate in limb-threatening and life-threatening ischemia. Although the risk is lower with LMWHs, both unfractionated heparin and LMWHs are associated with the development of HIT. HIT must be distinguished from transient early decreases in the platelet count that frequently normalize within 3 days despite ongoing administration of heparin. A decrease in the platelet count of greater than 50 % of baseline or a new thromboembolic event in the setting of any heparin product, including heparin flushes and heparin-coated catheters, should raise concern for true HIT and lead to the discontinuation of all heparin-containing products.

A clinical scoring system that incorporates the "4T's" can be used to evaluate patients in whom HIT is suspected: Thrombocytopenia, Timing, Thrombosis, and the absence of other more likely diagnoses (Table 9.2) [20]. Patients with a score of less than or equal to 3 have a low likelihood of HIT (<5 %). A score of 4 or 5 corresponds with an intermediate likelihood of HIT. Scores of 6 or greater indicate that HIT is likely (>80 %). HIT typically occurs within 4–14 days from initial heparin exposure but may occur earlier if the patient has been previously exposed to heparin. Clinicians should consider the diagnosis of delayed-onset HIT [21]. Antiplatelet factor 4/heparin antibody and serotonin release assay testing are the laboratory tests used to diagnose HIT. Higher levels of anti-platelet factor 4/heparin antibody are associated with increased risk of thrombosis among patients with clinically suspected HIT [22].

Table 9.2 A generally-accepted tool for assessing the probability of heparin-induced thrombocytopenia (HIT)

| | Points assigned for each category | | |
	2	1	0
Thrombocytopenia	>50 % platelet fall or nadir is 20×10^9/L	30–50 % platelet fall or nadir $10–19 \times 10^9$/L	<30 % platelet fall or nadir <10×10^9/L
Timing of onset of platelet drop or clinical sequelae	Fall between days 5–10 after initial heparin exposure, or within 1 day of heparin reexposure (if previous heparin exposure was within past 30 days)	Fall after day 10 or if timing unclear or within 1 day of heparin reexposure (if previous heparin exposure was within past 30–100 days)	Fall before day 5 and no recent heparin
Thrombosis or other sequelae	New proven thrombosis; skin necrosis; acute systemic reaction	Progressive or recurrent thrombosis; erythematous skin lesions; suspected thrombosis (not proven)	None
Other causes of platelet decline	None evident	Possible	Definite
"High probability" 6–8 points			
"Intermediate probability" 4–5 points			
"Low probability" 0–3 points			

When HIT is confirmed or even suspected, a direct thrombin inhibitor such as argatroban or bivalirudin should be administered. Unlike bivalirudin, argatroban does not require dose adjustment for renal insufficiency. However, argatroban is hepatically cleared and should be used with caution in patients with impaired liver function. Several other pitfalls in the management of HIT must be avoided. Warfarin as monotherapy should not be used for anticoagulation because it may worsen the procoagulant state and precipitate limb gangrene. Platelet transfusions "add more fuel to the fire" and are contraindicated. Inferior vena cava filter insertion without concomitant anticoagulation can result in caval, pelvic, and lower extremity venous thrombosis. LMWHs, although less likely to cause HIT, will often cross-react with IgG antibodies once HIT has developed and may lead to worsening thrombocytopenia and thrombosis.

Fondaparinux

Fondaparinux is a synthetic pentasaccharide with anti-Xa activity approved by the FDA for the initial therapy of DVT and PE. Fondaparinux has been shown to be at least as safe and effective as enoxaparin in the initial treatment of patients with symptomatic DVT [23]. Among hemodynamically stable patients with acute symptomatic PE, fondaparinux is as safe and effective as IV unfractionated heparin [24]. Fondaparinux is administered as a once-daily subcutaneous injection in fixed doses of 5 mg for body weight less than 50 kg, 7.5 mg for body weight of 50–100 kg, and 10 mg for body weight greater than 100 kg. Fondaparinux does not require routine monitoring or dose adjustment with laboratory coagulation tests. Because it is cleared by the kidneys, fondaparinux is contraindicated in patients with severe renal impairment. In contrast to unfractionated heparin and LMWH, fondaparinux does not cause HIT. Fondaparinux at a dose of 2.5 mg once daily for 45 days has been shown to be safe and effective in the treatment of patients with acute, symptomatic superficial vein thrombosis of the lower extremities [25]. However, there is no antidote or reversal agent to manage bleeding complications.

Oral Anticoagulation

Warfarin

Until the introduction of the NOACs, oral vitamin K antagonists such as warfarin had been the default agent for outpatient anticoagulation for VTE. Although a growing number of patients with VTE are being prescribed NOACs, warfarin remains an important option in the anticoagulation armamentarium. Oral anticoagulation is started concurrently with heparin, LMWH, or fondaparinux and overlapped for a minimum of 5 days until full therapeutic efficacy has been achieved. For the majority of patients with VTE, the target International Normalized Ratio (INR) is between 2.0 and 3.0. The majority of patients achieve a therapeutic INR with initial warfarin doses of 5 mg daily.

Management of warfarin anticoagulation can frequently be challenging because of many drug-food, drug-alcohol, and drug-drug interactions. Commonly implicated warfarin potentiators include acetaminophen, quinolone antibiotics, amiodarone, and antiplatelet agents such as clopidogrel. A subset of patients possess a genetic mutation in cytochrome P450 2C9 that leads to very slow metabolism of warfarin with low maintenance doses such as 1–2 mg daily to achieve a target INR between 2.0 and 3.0 [26, 27]. Polymorphisms in the gene encoding vitamin K epoxide reductase complex 1 (VKORC1) have also been demonstrated to impact the response to warfarin [28]. Dosing algorithms that incorporate pharmacogenetic testing have not improved the safety and efficacy of warfarin anticoagulation in large randomized controlled trials [29–31].

Anticoagulation management services utilize the expertise of pharmacists, nurses, nurse practitioners, physician assistants, and physician directors to manage the oral anticoagulation of large populations of anticoagulated patients. Such services facilitate the INR testing, dose adjustment, and clinical monitoring of patients of patients prescribed warfarin for oral anticoagulation. Anticoagulation management services play a critical role in maintaining the continuum of care from the inpatient to outpatient setting. Self-monitoring and, in appropriately selected patients, self-management of oral anticoagulation are safe options for further simplifying oral anticoagulation with warfarin [32].

Non-vitamin K Oral Anticoagulants (NOACs)

NOACs offer several advantages over warfarin for oral anticoagulation in patients with VTE (Table 9.3). Under routine conditions, NOACs do not require laboratory monitoring or dose adjustment, in contrast to warfarin, which requires careful INR monitoring and dose adjustment. While warfarin takes several days to achieve a therapeutic INR when initiating anticoagulation and 5–7 days to wear off when stopping anticoagulation, NOACs have a rapid onset of action and short half-life. NOACs also avoid the many drug-drug and drug-food interactions that complicate warfarin management. Medication adherence is imperative with the NOACs because of their short half-lives. In contrast to warfarin therapy in which the INR may remain therapeutic despite a missed dose or two, therapeutic anticoagulation with NOACs

Table 9.3 Major differences between the warfarin and the non-vitamin K oral anticoagulants (NOACs)

Feature	Warfarin	NOAC
Onset of action	Slow	Rapid
Dosing	Variable	Fixed
Drug-food effect	Yes	No
Drug-drug interactions	Many	Few
Routine laboratory monitoring	Yes	No
Half-life	Long	Short
Reversal agent	Yes	Not yet

is lost soon after an omitted dose. All of the NOACs are, at least in part, cleared renally. Conventional laboratory tests of coagulation such as the prothrombin time (PT), INR, or aPTT do not accurately measure the degree of anticoagulation in patients taking NOACs and should not be obtained.

Dabigatran, rivaroxaban, apixaban, and edoxaban have been shown to be safe and effective for oral anticoagulation for VTE and are all U.S. FDA approved. There is limited clinical trial experience with the NOACs in patients with severe thrombophilia and active cancer. Dabigatran and edoxaban are administered in fixed doses after at least 5 days of parenteral anticoagulation with unfractionated heparin, LMWHs, fondaparinux, or a direct thrombin inhibitor. Rivaroxaban and apixaban are administered as completely oral monotherapy, with a fixed loading dose followed by a maintenance dose. The patient in the Clinical Vignette elected to take a NOAC to avoid the need for routine laboratory monitoring and dose adjustment and because of the enhanced safety, in particular, the reduced risk of major bleeding complications.

Dabigatran

In a randomized, double-blind, noninferiority trial (RE-COVER) of 2539 patients with acute VTE who were initially given parenteral anticoagulation therapy, the oral direct thrombin inhibitor dabigatran (150 mg twice daily) was compared with dose-adjusted warfarin [6]. The primary study outcome was the 6-month incidence of recurrent symptomatic, objectively confirmed VTE and VTE-related death. Recurrent VTE was observed in 2.4 % of the patients randomized to dabigatran compared with 2.1 % of those randomized to warfarin ($p < 0.001$ for the prespecified noninferiority margin). Major bleeding occurred in 1.6 % of patients assigned to dabigatran and 1.9 % of those assigned to warfarin (HR with dabigatran, 0.82; 95 % confidence interval [CI], 0.45–1.48). Any bleeding was observed in 16.1 % of patients assigned to dabigatran and 21.9 % of those assigned to warfarin (HR with dabigatran, 0.71; 95 % CI, 0.59–0.85).

A second randomized, double-blind study (RE-COVER II) of 2568 patients with acute VTE who had been treated with LMWH for 5–11 days compared dabigatran (150 mg twice daily) with dose adjusted warfarin [5]. Over 6 months, 30 of 1279 patients randomized to dabigatran and 28 of 1289 patients randomized to warfarin experienced recurrent VTE (2.4 % vs. 2.2 %; HR, 1.08; 95 % CI, −1.0 to 1.5, $p < 0.0001$ for the pre-specified non-inferiority margin). Major bleeding occurred in 15 patients assigned to dabigatran and 22 assigned to warfarin (HR 0.69; 95 % CI, 0.56–0.81).

Rivaroxaban

A randomized noninferiority study (EINSTEIN-DVT) compared oral rivaroxaban (a factor Xa inhibitor) alone (15 mg twice daily for 3 weeks, followed by 20 mg once daily) with enoxaparin followed by a vitamin K antagonist in 3449 patients with acute, symptomatic DVT [2]. Rivaroxaban demonstrated noninferior efficacy compared with enoxaparin as a "bridge" to oral anticoagulation with a vitamin K antagonist with respect to the primary outcome of recurrent VTE (36 events [2.1 %], vs. 51 events [3.0 %]; HR, 0.68; 95 % CI, 0.44–1.04; p < 0.001). The rate of major bleeding or clinically relevant nonmajor bleeding was similar in both groups. In a second phase of the study in which rivaroxaban was compared with placebo for an additional 6 or 12 months in patients who had completed an initial 6–12 months of treatment for VTE, rivaroxaban had superior efficacy (8 events [1.3 %], vs. 42 with placebo [7.1 %]; HR, 0.18; 95 % CI, 0.09–0.39; p < 0.001).

A subsequent randomized noninferiority trial (EINSTEIN-PE) of 4832 patients who had acute symptomatic PE with or without DVT compared rivaroxaban (15 mg twice daily for 3 weeks, followed by 20 mg once daily) with standard therapy with enoxaparin followed by a dose-adjusted vitamin K antagonist [4]. Rivaroxaban was noninferior to standard therapy (noninferiority margin, 2.0; p = 0.003) for the primary efficacy outcome of symptomatic recurrent VTE (2.1 % versus 1.8 % in the standard-therapy group) (HR, 1.12; 95 % CI, 0.75–1.68). Major bleeding was observed in 1.1 % of the rivaroxaban group versus 2.2 % of the standard-therapy group (HR, 0.49; 95 % CI, 0.31–0.79; p = 0.003).

Apixaban

In a randomized, double-blind study (AMPLIFY), another factor Xa inhibitor, apixaban (administered as a loading dose of 10 mg twice daily for 7 days, followed by 5 mg twice daily) was compared with subcutaneously-administered enoxaparin followed by warfarin in 5395 patients with acute venous thromboembolism [1]. The primary efficacy outcome of recurrent symptomatic VTE or VTE-related death occurred in 59 of 2609 patients (2.3 %) in the apixaban group compared with 71 of 2635 (2.7 %) in the warfarin group (relative risk, 0.84; 95 % CI, 0.60–1.18; p < 0.001 for non-inferiority). Major bleeding occurred in 0.6 % of patients who received apixaban and in 1.8 % of those who warfarin (relative risk, 0.31; 95 % CI, 0.17–0.55; p < 0.001 for superiority). A composite outcome of major bleeding and clinically relevant nonmajor bleeding occurred in 4.3 % of the patients in the apixaban group compared with 9.7 % of those in the conventional-therapy group (relative risk, 0.44; 95 % CI, 0.36–0.55; p < 0.001).

Edoxaban

Edoxaban, another factor Xa inhibitor, was evaluated in the HOKUSAI-VTE study which compared parenteral anticoagulation (unfractionated heparin or LMWH) followed by edoxaban with parenteral anticoagulation followed by warfarin in 8292 patients with DVT, PE, or both [3]. Recurrence of symptomatic VTE occurred in 3.2 % of patients in the edoxaban group and 3.5 % in the warfarin group (HR, 0.89; 95 % CI, 0.7–1.13; p < 0.001 for non-inferiority). Clinically relevant bleeding (major and non-major) occurred in 8.5 % of patients in the edoxaban group and 10.3 % in the warfarin group (HR, 0.81; 95 % CI, 0.71–0.94; p=0.004 for superiority). The difference in the primary safety outcome was largely because of a reduction in clinically relevant non-major bleeding. Among a prespecified group of patients with "severe PE" with evidence of RV dysfunction (NT-proBNP ≥500 pg/mL), recurrent symptomatic VTE occurred in 3.3 % of patients in the edoxaban group and 6.2 % in the warfarin group (HR, 0.52; 95 % CI, 0.28–0.98).

Management of Oral Anticoagulant Associated-Bleeding

Warfarin

In the event of minor excessive oral anticoagulation without active bleeding, one or two doses of warfarin should be held, and the INR should be rechecked serially until it falls within the therapeutic range. In asymptomatic patients with supertherapeutic INRs between 5.0 and 9.0, vitamin K more rapidly reverses INR, but does not decrease major bleeding. Vitamin K should be reserved for asymptomatic patients with INR greater than 10, or in special patient populations with supertherapeutic INRs (advanced age, heart failure, malignancy) [33]. Four-factor prothrombin-complex concentrate (PCC) is preferred to reverse excessive oral anticoagulation in the setting of active bleeding [34]. Concomitant intravenous vitamin K should be administered to prevent "rebound" anticoagulation once the effect of PCC has worn off.

Non-vitamin K Oral Anticoagulants

NOAC-associated minor bleeding is best managed by local measures, such as compression, and holding anticoagulation until hemostasis is achieved and the source of the bleed has been addressed. Severe or life-threatening bleeding associated with NOAC administration should focus on enhancing elimination with activated charcoal (if last dose within 2 h) or urgent hemodialysis followed by activated PCC for dabigatran and four-factor PCC for the direct factor Xa inhibitors [35]. Specific reversal agents, including a monoclonal antibody fragment for dabigatran [36] and a recombinant factor Xa derivative for the direct Xa inhibitors [37], are being evaluated in the clinical trial setting and may be available in the near future.

Tips for Outpatient Anticoagulation

Management of outpatient anticoagulation with warfarin can challenge even the most experienced healthcare providers. Several important interventions such as the use of patient-centered educational materials and centralized anticoagulation clinics may help avoid many of the management pitfalls of outpatient anticoagulation therapy (Table 9.4). The frequent need for laboratory visits for INR testing may

Table 9.4 Tips for management of outpatient anticoagulation with warfarin

Insist on detailed and explicit communication between all of the patient's healthcare providers and clearly designate who will manage the anticoagulation
Clearly explain to the patient and family the rationale for anticoagulation and the major risks from supertherapeutic (bleeding) and subtherapeutic levels (thromboembolism)
Define the relationship between important terms such as prothrombin time, International Normalized Ratio (INR), and dose adjustment of the anticoagulant
Use a software-supported electronic surveillance system that will keep track of prior anticoagulation levels and flag patients in whom an expected laboratory value has not been reported
Consider the use of centralized anticoagulation clinics
Avoid warfarin dose adjustments of greater than 20 % of the previous dose
Changes in the INR are most reflective of the warfarin dose given 3–5 days prior

Table 9.5 Factors to consider when selecting a non-vitamin K oral anticoagulant (NOAC)

Factor	Rivaroxaban	Dabigatran	Apixaban	Edoxaban
Dosing	Initiation: 15 mg twice daily for 3 weeks Maintenance: 20 mg daily	Initiation: Use parenteral anticoagulation for 5–10 days Maintenance: 150 mg twice daily	Initiation: 10 mg twice daily for 7 days Maintenance: 5 mg twice daily Long-term prevention after at least 6 months: 2.5 mg twice daily	Initiation: Use parenteral anticoagulation for 5–10 days Maintenance: 60 mg daily
Renal clearance	33 %	80 %	25 %	35 %
Maintenance dose adjustment	No adjustment if CrCl ≥30 mL/min Avoid use if CrCl <30 mL/min	No adjustment if CrCl >30 mL/min Avoid use if CrCl ≤30 mL/min	No adjustment if CrCl ≥25 mL/min Avoid use if CrCl <25 mL/min	30 mg daily if weight ≤60 kg

CrCl creatinine clearance

represent a minor inconvenience for some patients and a major limitation to quality of life in others. Home INR monitoring and warfarin self-management may be safe alternatives in appropriately selected patients [32]. NOACs have the potential to facilitate outpatient anticoagulation by eliminating the need for routine laboratory monitoring and frequent dose adjustment. Selection of a NOAC should consider dosing frequency, renal clearance, and parameters for dose reduction (Table 9.5). Although prices have decreased since their introduction into the marketplace, NOACs cost more than warfarin. However, depending on their prescription plan, patients may fill NOAC prescriptions at a reduced cost through manufacturer-sponsored co-pay assistance plans. The financial burden of the particular agent, the lifestyle impact of INR testing, and patient preference should be weighed in selection of the optimal agent for anticoagulation.

Answer Key

1. **Correct answer**, (**a**) LMWHs such as dalteparin are preferred for treatment of VTE in patients with active malignancy because they halve the risk of recurrence compared with warfarin. Dabigatran is largely renally-cleared and should not be used in hemodialysis patients. Oral anticoagulation, with warfarin or a NOAC, is not recommended for patients in whom enteric absorption is abnormal. LMWHs should not be used in patients with suspected or confirmed HIT because they will, like other heparin compounds, cross-react with the heparin-platelet factor 4 antibodies.
2. **Correct answer**, (**b**) NOACs are non-inferior with regard to efficacy and superior with regard to bleeding complications compared with warfarin. Despite reductions in price, NOACs are still more expensive than warfarin. Medication adherence is a critical consideration in patient considering NOACs because missed doses result in rapid loss of anticoagulant effect. Apixaban and rivaroxaban, not edoxaban, are approved for completely oral monotherapy.
3. **Correct answer**, (**c**) Hemodialysis is helpful for eliminating circulating dabigatran, not apixaban, in patients with overdose or severe or life-threatening bleeding.

References

1. Agnelli G, Buller HR, Cohen A, et al. Oral apixaban for the treatment of acute venous thromboembolism. N Engl J Med. 2013;369:799–808.
2. Bauersachs R, Berkowitz SD, Brenner B, et al. Oral rivaroxaban for symptomatic venous thromboembolism. N Engl J Med. 2010;363:2499–510.
3. Buller HR, Decousus H, Grosso MA, et al. Edoxaban versus warfarin for the treatment of symptomatic venous thromboembolism. N Engl J Med. 2013;369:1406–15.
4. Buller HR, Prins MH, Lensin AW, et al. Oral rivaroxaban for the treatment of symptomatic pulmonary embolism. N Engl J Med. 2012;366:1287–97.
5. Schulman S, Kakkar AK, Goldhaber SZ, et al. Treatment of acute venous thromboembolism with dabigatran or warfarin and pooled analysis. Circulation. 2014;129:764–72.
6. Schulman S, Kearon C, Kakkar AK, et al. Dabigatran versus warfarin in the treatment of acute venous thromboembolism. N Engl J Med. 2009;361:2342–52.
7. Raschke R, Hirsh J, Guidry JR. Suboptimal monitoring and dosing of unfractionated heparin in comparative studies with low-molecular-weight heparin. Ann Intern Med. 2003;138:720–3.
8. Raschke RA, Reilly BM, Guidry JR, Fontana JR, Srinivas S. The weight-based heparin dosing nomogram compared with a "standard care" nomogram. A randomized controlled trial. Ann Intern Med. 1993;119:874–81.
9. Piazza G, Goldhaber SZ. Fibrinolysis for acute pulmonary embolism. Vasc Med. 2010;15:419–28.

10. Breddin HK, Hach-Wunderle V, Nakov R, Kakkar VV. Effects of a low-molecular-weight heparin on thrombus regression and recurrent thromboembolism in patients with deep-vein thrombosis. N Engl J Med. 2001;344:626–31.
11. Gould MK, Dembitzer AD, Doyle RL, Hastie TJ, Garber AM. Low-molecular-weight heparins compared with unfractionated heparin for treatment of acute deep venous thrombosis. A meta-analysis of randomized, controlled trials. Ann Intern Med. 1999;130:800–9.
12. Merli G, Spiro TE, Olsson CG, et al. Subcutaneous enoxaparin once or twice daily compared with intravenous unfractionated heparin for treatment of venous thromboembolic disease. Ann Intern Med. 2001;134:191–202.
13. Low-molecular-weight heparin in the treatment of patients with venous thromboembolism. The Columbus Investigators. N Engl J Med. 1997;337:657–62.
14. Simonneau G, Sors H, Charbonnier B, et al. A comparison of low-molecular-weight heparin with unfractionated heparin for acute pulmonary embolism. The THESEE Study Group. Tinzaparine ou Heparine Standard: Evaluations dans l'Embolie Pulmonaire. N Engl J Med. 1997;337:663–9.
15. Jaff MR, McMurtry MS, Archer SL, et al. Management of massive and submassive pulmonary embolism, iliofemoral deep vein thrombosis, and chronic thromboembolic pulmonary hypertension: a scientific statement from the American Heart Association. Circulation. 2011;123:1788–830.
16. Kearon C, Akl EA, Comerota AJ, et al. Antithrombotic therapy for VTE disease: antithrombotic therapy and prevention of thrombosis, 9th ed: American College of Chest Physicians Evidence-Based Clinical Practice Guidelines. Chest. 2012;141:e419S–94.
17. Lee AY, Levine MN, Baker RI, et al. Low-molecular-weight heparin versus a coumarin for the prevention of recurrent venous thromboembolism in patients with cancer. N Engl J Med. 2003;349:146–53.
18. Bounameaux H, de Moerloose P. Is laboratory monitoring of low-molecular-weight heparin therapy necessary? No. J Thromb Haemost. 2004;2:551–4.
19. Harenberg J. Is laboratory monitoring of low-molecular-weight heparin therapy necessary? Yes. J Thromb Haemost. 2004;2:547–50.
20. Warkentin TE, Greinacher A, Koster A, Lincoff AM, American College of Chest P. Treatment and prevention of heparin-induced thrombocytopenia: American College of Chest Physicians Evidence-Based Clinical Practice Guidelines (8th Edition). Chest. 2008;133:340S–80.
21. Rice L, Attisha WK, Drexler A, Francis JL. Delayed-onset heparin-induced thrombocytopenia. Ann Intern Med. 2002;136:210–5.
22. Baroletti S, Hurwitz S, Conti NA, Fanikos J, Piazza G, Goldhaber SZ. Thrombosis in suspected heparin-induced thrombocytopenia occurs more often with high antibody levels. Am J Med. 2012;125:44–9.
23. Buller HR, Davidson BL, Decousus H, et al. Fondaparinux or enoxaparin for the initial treatment of symptomatic deep venous thrombosis: a randomized trial. Ann Intern Med. 2004;140:867–73.
24. Buller HR, Davidson BL, Decousus H, et al. Subcutaneous fondaparinux versus intravenous unfractionated heparin in the initial treatment of pulmonary embolism. N Engl J Med. 2003;349:1695–702.
25. Decousus H, Prandoni P, Mismetti P, et al. Fondaparinux for the treatment of superficial-vein thrombosis in the legs. N Engl J Med. 2010;363:1222–32.
26. Higashi MK, Veenstra DL, Kondo LM, et al. Association between CYP2C9 genetic variants and anticoagulation-related outcomes during warfarin therapy. JAMA. 2002;287:1690–8.
27. Joffe HV, Xu R, Johnson FB, Longtine J, Kucher N, Goldhaber SZ. Warfarin dosing and cytochrome P450 2C9 polymorphisms. Thromb Haemost. 2004;91:1123–8.
28. Rieder MJ, Reiner AP, Gage BF, et al. Effect of VKORC1 haplotypes on transcriptional regulation and warfarin dose. N Engl J Med. 2005;352:2285–93.
29. Kimmel SE, French B, Kasner SE, et al. A pharmacogenetic versus a clinical algorithm for warfarin dosing. N Engl J Med. 2013;369:2283–93.
30. Pirmohamed M, Burnside G, Eriksson N, et al. A randomized trial of genotype-guided dosing of warfarin. N Engl J Med. 2013;369:2294–303.

31. Verhoef TI, Ragia G, de Boer A, et al. A randomized trial of genotype-guided dosing of aceno-coumarol and phenprocoumon. N Engl J Med. 2013;369:2304–12.
32. Heneghan C, Ward A, Perera R, et al. Self-monitoring of oral anticoagulation: systematic review and meta-analysis of individual patient data. Lancet. 2012;379:322–34.
33. Garcia DA, Crowther MA. Reversal of warfarin: case-based practice recommendations. Circulation. 2012;125:2944–7.
34. Deveras RA, Kessler CM. Reversal of warfarin-induced excessive anticoagulation with recombinant human factor VIIa concentrate. Ann Intern Med. 2002;137:884–8.
35. Siegal DM, Crowther MA. Acute management of bleeding in patients on novel oral anticoagulants. Eur Heart J. 2013;34:489–98b.
36. Pollack CV, Reilly PA, Eikelboom J, et al. Idarucizumab for Dabigatran Reversal. N Engl J Med. 2015 Jun 22. [Epub ahead of print].
37. Lu G, DeGuzman FR, Hollenbach SJ, et al. A specific antidote for reversal of anticoagulation by direct and indirect inhibitors of coagulation factor Xa. Nat Med. 2013;19:446–51.

Chapter 10
Long-Term Management of Venous Thromboembolism: Strategies for Reducing the Risk of Recurrence

Abstract Long-term care of patients with venous thromboembolism (VTE) includes determining the optimal duration of anticoagulation after VTE. Selection of the optimal duration and drug regimen requires an individualized assessment of the patient's long-term risk of recurrence as well as bleeding. Warfarin and non-vitamin K oral anticoagulants (NOACs) have been validated for extended duration anticoagulation to prevent recurrent unprovoked VTE. Aspirin also plays a role in the prevention of recurrence in patients with unprovoked VTE.

Keywords Aspirin • Duration of anticoagulation • NOACs • Venous thromboembolism recurrence • Warfarin

Self-Assessment Questions

1. Which of the following oral regimens has not been proven to decrease the long-term risk of recurrent VTE in patients with an initial unprovoked pulmonary embolism (PE) or deep vein thrombosis (DVT) who have completed an initial 6–12 months of anticoagulation?

   (a) Warfarin with an International Normalized Ratio (INR) intensity of 1.5–2.0
   (b) Warfarin with an INR intensity of 2.0–3.0
   (c) Apixaban 2.5 mg twice daily
   (d) Edoxaban 60 mg once daily
   (e) Aspirin 100 mg orally daily

2. Extended duration anticoagulation to prevent a high risk of VTE recurrence should be prescribed to which of the following patients?

   (a) A 25-year-old woman who developed bilateral PE and right-sided DVT in the setting of a combination oral contraceptive pill
   (b) A 89-year-old woman with a history of rheumatoid arthritis and recurrent diverticular bleeding who developed unprovoked bilateral PE
   (c) A 72-year-old man with a history of obesity who developed an unprovoked left calf DVT
   (d) A 55-year-old woman with factor V Leiden heterozygosity who developed right-sided PE in the setting of estrogen-based hormone replacement therapy

© Springer International Publishing Switzerland 2015
G. Piazza et al., *Handbook for Venous Thromboembolism*,
DOI 10.1007/978-3-319-20843-5_10

Clinical Vignette

A 67-year-old man with history of hypertension and diabetes presented with progressive left leg swelling and calf discomfort. He denied any recent trauma, major surgery, or periods of immobility. He initially attributed the discomfort to an increase in his exercise routine. However, after it persisted despite a hiatus from exercise, he presented to his Primary Care Physician. A venous ultrasound was performed and documented left popliteal DVT (Fig. 10.1). The patient was treated with rivaroxaban 15 mg orally twice daily for 3 weeks and then 20 mg daily thereafter for a total of 6 months of anticoagulation. Six months after discontinuing rivaroxaban, he developed recurrent left leg swelling and discomfort this time involving the whole lower extremity. Again, he noted no recent trauma, major surgery, or immobility. The pain was so severe that the patient was having difficulty ambulating. He presented to the Emergency Department where he was noted to have a tender and tensely edematous left thigh and calf. Venous ultrasound demonstrated new left common femoral and femoral deep vein thrombosis (Figs. 10.2 and 10.3). Because of the severity of his symptoms, Vascular Medicine was consulted and recommended catheter-directed fibrinolysis. The patient noted marked improvement in his lower extremity symptoms following overnight catheter-based fibrinolysis. May-Thurner compression was not observed on repeat venography the following day. He was restarted on rivaroxaban 15 mg twice daily for 3 weeks followed 20 mg daily thereafter. He was referred to Vascular Medicine clinic after hospital discharge to determine the optimal duration of anticoagulation. His Vascular Medicine physician recommended extended duration anticoagulation with rivaroxaban 20 mg daily because of the patient's recurrent unprovoked DVTs and high risk for recurrence.

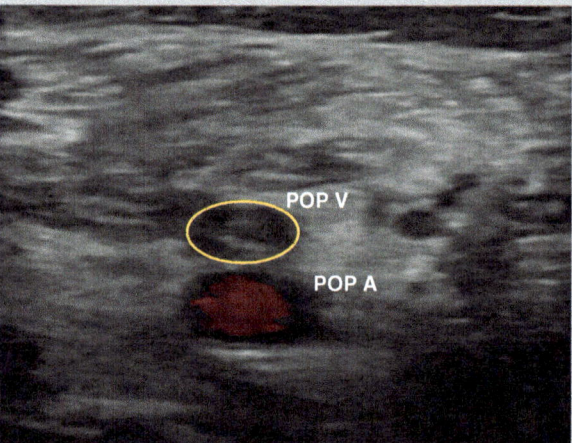

Fig. 10.1 Venous ultrasound demonstrating echogenic material (*oval*) in the left popliteal vein (*POP V*) consistent with acute deep vein thrombosis (DVT) in a 67-year-old man with history of hypertension and diabetes who presented with progressive left leg swelling and calf discomfort. In contrast to the left popliteal artery (*POP A*), there is no evidence of color Doppler flow in the left popliteal vein because it has thrombosed

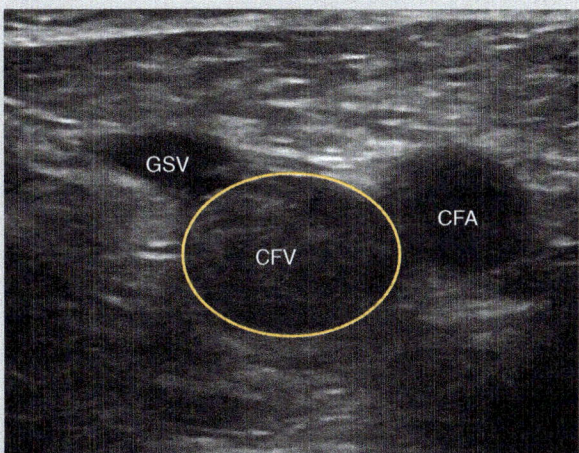

Fig. 10.2 Venous ultrasound demonstrating echogenic material (*oval*) in a dilated left common femoral vein (*CFV*) consistent with acute deep vein thrombosis (DVT) in a 67-year-old man with history of hypertension, diabetes, and prior DVT who presented with severe entire left leg swelling and discomfort. The left greater saphenous vein (*GSV*) and common femoral artery (*CFA*) appear normal

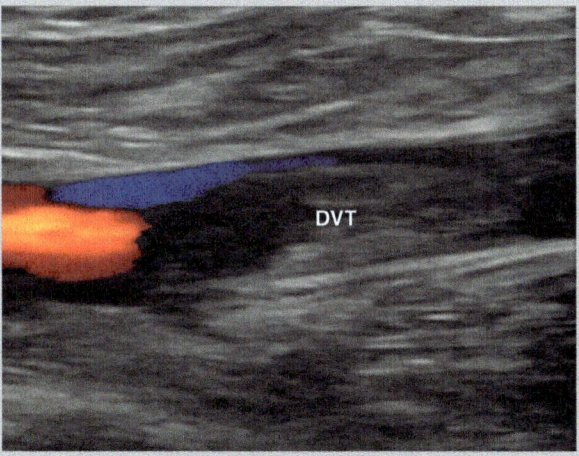

Fig. 10.3 Venous ultrasound demonstrating a large amount of echogenic material in the left common femoral vein with a small residual channel of color Doppler flow consistent with nearly totally occlusive deep vein thrombosis (*DVT*) in a 67-year-old man with history of hypertension, diabetes, and prior DVT who presented with severe entire left leg swelling and discomfort

Optimal Duration of Anticoagulation

Determining the optimal duration of anticoagulation after VTE requires an individualized assessment of the patient's long-term risk of recurrence as well as bleeding (Fig. 10.4) [1, 2]. A population-based strategy recommends time-limited anticoagulation of 3–6 months for provoked VTE and extended duration anticoagulation for patients with low bleeding risk and unprovoked (idiopathic) VTE. The patient in the Clinical Vignette provides an example of a patient with an initial unprovoked DVT who was prescribed only time-limited (6 months) of anticoagulation who subsequently developed an extensive recurrent unprovoked DVT. The patient would have benefited from extended duration anticoagulation following the initial event and was ultimately prescribed long-term therapy with rivaroxaban after the second unprovoked DVT.

Patients with VTE in the setting of malignancy have an increased risk of recurrent VTE and are generally prescribed extended duration anticoagulation with a LMWH as long as they have active cancer [3]. Similarly, VTE patients with severe thrombophilia, such as those with antiphospholipid antibodies, deficiencies of protein C, S, or antithrombin, or homozygosity for factor V Leiden or the prothrombin gene mutation, are often prescribed extended duration anticoagulation because of a high risk of recurrence. Although not endorsed by published evidence-based guidelines, a patient-specific strategy utilizing D-dimer testing or lower extremity venous imaging after completion of standard anticoagulation for VTE has been evaluated to determine optimal duration of anticoagulation [4]. However, a prospective clinical study found that the risk for recurrence in patients with a first unprovoked VTE who had negative D-dimer results was not low enough to justify stopping anticoagulation [5]. Other chronic medical conditions that predispose to VTE, such as chronic obstructive pulmonary disease, heart failure, systemic inflammatory disorders, and

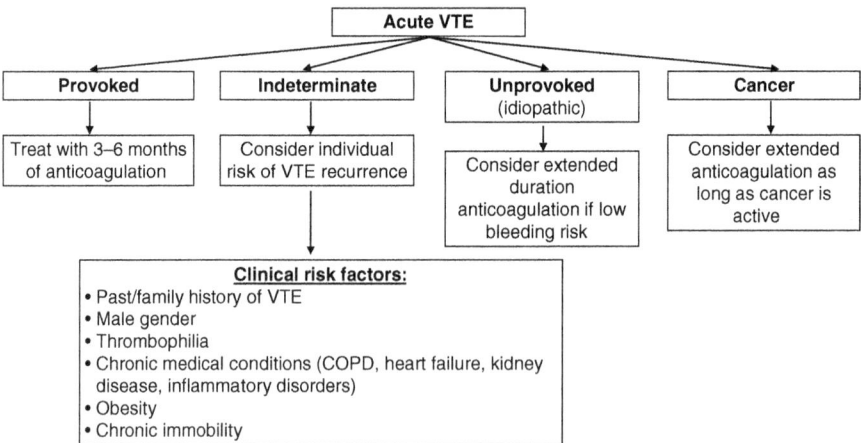

Fig. 10.4 An approach to optimizing duration of anticoagulation in patients with venous thromboembolism (*VTE*). *COPD* chronic obstructive pulmonary disease

obesity, may also be considered in the decision-making regarding optimal duration of anticoagulation [1].

Warfarin and NOACs have been validated for extended duration anticoagulation to prevent recurrent unprovoked VTE. In the PREVENT study, a double-blind, randomized, controlled trial of 508 unprovoked VTE patients who had completed an average of 6 months of full-intensity warfarin, extended duration anticoagulation with low-intensity warfarin (target INR of 1.5–2) for an average of 2 years reduced the recurrence rate by two-thirds compared with placebo [6]. Low-intensity warfarin was highly effective in preventing recurrent VTE in all subgroups, even in patients with factor V Leiden or the prothrombin gene mutation. In the ELATE study of 739 patients with unprovoked VTE, extended duration, full-intensity warfarin (target INR 2–3) was as safe as but more effective than extended duration, low-intensity warfarin therapy (target INR 1.5–1.9) [7].

Among the NOACs, rivaroxaban, dabigatran, and apixaban have shown to be safe and effective alternatives for long-term prevention of recurrent VTE in patients with an unprovoked (idiopathic) event [8–10]. The NOACs are associated with an 80–90 % reduction in relative risk of recurrent symptomatic VTE. The patient in the Clinical Vignette was treated with extended duration anticoagulation with rivaroxaban 20 mg orally daily.

Aspirin for Prevention of Recurrent Venous Thromboembolism

Aspirin may also play a role in the prevention of recurrence in patients with unprovoked VTE. In a multicenter, investigator-initiated, double-blind study, patients with an initial unprovoked VTE who had completed 6–18 months of oral anticoagulant treatment were randomly assigned to aspirin, 100 mg daily, or placebo for 2 years [11]. VTE recurred in 28 of the 205 patients who received aspirin and in 43 of the 197 patients who received placebo (6.6 % vs. 11.2 % per year; hazard ratio [HR], 0.58; 95 % confidence interval [CI], 0.36–0.93). One patient in each treatment group had a major bleeding event.

A second multicenter, double-blind study compared aspirin, 100 mg daily, with placebo for 2 years [12]. Eight hundred and twenty two patients who had been prescribed initial anticoagulation for between 6 weeks and 24 months were enrolled in the trial. Recurrent VTE occurred in 57 of 411 patients assigned to aspirin and in 73 of 411 patients assigned to placebo (4.8 % vs. 6.5 % per year; HR, 0.74; 95 % CI, 0.52–1.05, $p=0.09$). The rate of VTE, myocardial infarction, stroke, major bleeding, or death from any cause was reduced by 33 % in the aspirin group (HR, 0.67; 95 % CI, 0.49–0.91, $p=0.01$) and demonstrated a net clinical benefit.

A meta-analysis of these trials of low-dose aspirin versus placebo in patients who completed standard anticoagulation for first unprovoked VTE demonstrated a 35 % relative risk reduction in recurrent VTE, a 37 % relative risk reduction in major vascular events, an overall net clinical benefit, and no increased risk of major bleeding [13].

Lifestyle Modification

While patient education about cardiovascular risk modification is standard of care for those hospitalized with myocardial infarction or stroke, it has only recently been recognized as a critical component of VTE management. VTE shares important risk factors with atherosclerotic cardiovascular disease, including diabetes, hypertension, obesity, dyslipidemia, and smoking [14–16]. Atherosclerotic cardiovascular disease itself is associated with an increased risk of VTE [17, 18]. Reciprocally, prior history of VTE is associated with a higher rate of myocardial infarction [19] and stroke [20].

Lifestyle modification efforts to reduce the risk of recurrent VTE and other cardiovascular events such as myocardial infarction and stroke should focus on a heart healthy diet, regular aerobic exercise, weight reduction for overweight and obese patients, and tobacco cessation [17]. Similar to patients with coronary artery disease or atherosclerotic cerebrovascular disease, VTE patients should be counseled to reduce intake of red and processed meats and to increase consumption of fish, fruits, and vegetables in order to reduce the risk of disease recurrence [21]. Furthermore, cardiovascular risk factors of diabetes mellitus, hypertension, and dyslipidemia should be treated according to the goals set forth by evidence-based guideline recommendations.

Psychosocial Support

The diagnosis of VTE may result in significant psychological and emotional trauma. The disease may strike patients of any age who are often otherwise healthy and frequently carries lifelong implications for disease recurrence. PE support groups help patients understand that they are not alone and provide useful advice on how to cope with the disease and its management [22]. Patient advocacy groups, such as the North American Thrombosis Forum (www.NATFonline.org), provide patients, families, providers, and other health care professionals with educational materials and programs to encourage a greater understanding of VTE and foster disease prevention efforts.

Follow-Up After Venous Thromboembolism

VTE may be the harbinger of an occult cancer that will subsequently be diagnosed [23–25]. Age-appropriate cancer screening should be reviewed and updated as necessary, according to evidence-based practice guidelines in patients with a new diagnosis of VTE.

Answer Key

1. **Correct answer**, (**d**) Edoxaban was shown to be safe and effective for the initial anticoagulation of patients with acute VTE in the HOKUSAI-VTE study. Edoxaban has not been evaluated for extended duration anticoagulation to prevent recurrent events in patients with initial unprovoked DVT or PE.

2. **Correct answer**, (**c**) The 72-year-old man has increased risk of VTE recurrence on account of his obesity and unprovoked DVT. The 24-year-old woman and 55-year-old woman had provoked VTE and require 6 months of anticoagulation. Factor V Leiden heterozygosity is not an indication for extended duration anticoagulation. The 89-year-old woman with rheumatoid arthritis and unprovoked PE has a high risk of VTE recurrence but is also high risk for bleeding and accordingly is not a candidate for extended duration anticoagulation after completing 6 months of anticoagulant therapy.

References

1. Goldhaber SZ, Piazza G. Optimal duration of anticoagulation after venous thromboembolism. Circulation. 2011;123:664–7.
2. Kearon C, Akl EA, Comerota AJ, et al. Antithrombotic therapy for VTE disease: antithrombotic therapy and prevention of thrombosis, 9th ed: American College of Chest Physicians Evidence-Based Clinical Practice Guidelines. Chest. 2012;141:e419S–94.
3. Piazza G. Venous thromboembolism and cancer. Circulation. 2013;128:2614–8.
4. Palareti G, Cosmi B, Legnani C, et al. D-dimer testing to determine the duration of anticoagulation therapy. N Engl J Med. 2006;355:1780–9.
5. Kearon C, Spencer FA, O'Keeffe D, et al. D-dimer testing to select patients with a first unprovoked venous thromboembolism who can stop anticoagulant therapy: a cohort study. Ann Intern Med. 2015;162:27–34.
6. Ridker PM, Goldhaber SZ, Danielson E, et al. Long-term, low-intensity warfarin therapy for the prevention of recurrent venous thromboembolism. N Engl J Med. 2003;348:1425–34.
7. Kearon C, Ginsberg JS, Kovacs MJ, et al. Comparison of low-intensity warfarin therapy with conventional-intensity warfarin therapy for long-term prevention of recurrent venous thromboembolism. N Engl J Med. 2003;349:631–9.
8. Agnelli G, Buller HR, Cohen A, et al. Apixaban for extended treatment of venous thromboembolism. N Engl J Med. 2013;368:699–708.
9. Bauersachs R, Berkowitz SD, Brenner B, et al. Oral rivaroxaban for symptomatic venous thromboembolism. N Engl J Med. 2010;363:2499–510.
10. Schulman S, Kearon C, Kakkar AK, et al. Extended use of dabigatran, warfarin, or placebo in venous thromboembolism. N Engl J Med. 2013;368:709–18.
11. Becattini C, Agnelli G, Schenone A, et al. Aspirin for preventing the recurrence of venous thromboembolism. N Engl J Med. 2012;366:1959–67.
12. Brighton TA, Eikelboom JW, Mann K, et al. Low-dose aspirin for preventing recurrent venous thromboembolism. N Engl J Med. 2012;367:1979–87.
13. Simes J, Becattini C, Agnelli G, et al. Aspirin for the prevention of recurrent venous thromboembolism: the INSPIRE collaboration. Circulation. 2014;130:1062–71.

14. Ageno W, Becattini C, Brighton T, Selby R, Kamphuisen PW. Cardiovascular risk factors and venous thromboembolism: a meta-analysis. Circulation. 2008;117:93–102.
15. Parkin L, Sweetland S, Balkwill A, Green J, Reeves G, Beral V. Body mass index, surgery, and risk of venous thromboembolism in middle-aged women: a cohort study. Circulation. 2012;125:1897–904.
16. Rosengren A, Freden M, Hansson PO, Wilhelmsen L, Wedel H, Eriksson H. Psychosocial factors and venous thromboembolism: a long-term follow-up study of Swedish men. J Thromb Haemost. 2008;6:558–64.
17. Piazza G, Goldhaber SZ. Venous thromboembolism and atherothrombosis. Circulation. 2010;121:2146–50.
18. Prandoni P, Bilora F, Marchiori A, et al. An association between atherosclerosis and venous thrombosis. N Engl J Med. 2003;348:1435–41.
19. Spencer FA, Ginsberg JS, Chong A, Alter DA. The relationship between unprovoked venous thromboembolism, age, and acute myocardial infarction. J Thromb Haemost. 2008;6:1507–13.
20. Sorensen HT, Horvath-Puho E, Pedersen L, Baron JA, Prandoni P. Venous thromboembolism and subsequent hospitalisation due to acute arterial cardiovascular events: a 20-year cohort study. Lancet. 2007;370:1773–9.
21. Steffen LM, Folsom AR, Cushman M, Jacobs Jr DR, Rosamond WD. Greater fish, fruit, and vegetable intakes are related to lower incidence of venous thromboembolism: the Longitudinal Investigation of Thromboembolism Etiology. Circulation. 2007;115:188–95.
22. Goldhaber SZ, Morrison RB. Cardiology patient pages. Pulmonary embolism and deep vein thrombosis. Circulation. 2002;106:1436–8.
23. Douketis JD, Gu C, Piccioli A, Ghirarduzzi A, Pengo V, Prandoni P. The long-term risk of cancer in patients with a first episode of venous thromboembolism. J Thromb Haemost. 2009;7:546–51.
24. Sorensen HT, Johnsen SP. Venous thromboembolism and subsequent short-term risk of an occult cancer. J Thromb Haemost. 2008;6:249–50.
25. Trujillo-Santos J, Prandoni P, Rivron-Guillot K, et al. Clinical outcome in patients with venous thromboembolism and hidden cancer: findings from the RIETE Registry. J Thromb Haemost. 2008;6:251–5.

Chapter 11
Chronic Thromboembolic Pulmonary Hypertension: A Pathophysiologic Basis for Diagnosis and Management

Abstract Chronic thromboembolic pulmonary hypertension (CTEPH) may follow both single and recurrent episodes of pulmonary embolism (PE) and is characterized by persistent macrovascular obstruction, pulmonary vasoconstriction, and a secondary small-vessel arteriopathy. CTEPH used to be considered a rare complication but is now recognized to occur in 2–4 % of patients after PE. While patients may be initially asymptomatic, CTEPH frequently progresses to debilitating exercise intolerance, chronic dyspnea, and may culminate in chronic right ventricular (RV) failure. Pulmonary thromboendarterectomy is the most effective therapy for CTEPH. Pulmonary vasodilators offer patients with CTEPH who are inoperable and those with post-operative persistent or recurrent pulmonary hypertension the potential for improved symptoms and functional capacity.

Keywords Chronic thromboembolic pulmonary hypertension • Diagnosis • Pathophysiology • Treatment

Self-Assessment Questions

1. Which of the following is not a risk factor for CTEPH?

   (a) Antiphospholipid antibodies
   (b) Hyperthyroidism
   (c) Recurrent PE
   (d) Systemic fibrinolytic therapy for PE
   (e) Pulmonary artery systolic pressure of 50 mmHg 6 months after PE diagnosis

2. Which of the following is the definitive therapy for CTEPH?

   (a) Warfarin with a target INR of 2.0–3.0.
   (b) Riociguat 2.5 mg three-times daily
   (c) Surgical pulmonary thromboendarterectomy
   (d) Balloon pulmonary artery angioplasty and stenting

© Springer International Publishing Switzerland 2015
G. Piazza et al., *Handbook for Venous Thromboembolism*,
DOI 10.1007/978-3-319-20843-5_11

Clinical Vignette

A 69-year-old man with unprovoked PE 2 months prior was referred to Cardiovascular Medicine Clinic for exertional dyspnea despite consistently therapeutic anticoagulation with warfarin. Although the dyspnea and chest pressure associated with his diagnosis of PE improved initially with anticoagulation, these symptoms never resolved completely and became progressively worse. He had presented to his local Emergency Department 1 month earlier with chest pressure and dyspnea. A contrast-enhanced chest computed tomogram (CT) was performed and demonstrated no new PE. He was instructed to continue warfarin and follow-up with his Primary Care Physician, who subsequently referred him for cardiovascular evaluation. On physical examination, he had a heart rate of 105 beats per minute, blood pressure of 113/76 mmHg, respiratory rate of 22 breaths per minute, and an oxygen saturation of 90 % on room air. Although his lungs were clear to auscultation, his cardiac examination was remarkable for tachycardia, a loud sound of pulmonic closure (P2), and a III/VI holosystolic murmur at the left lower sternal border that increased with inspiration. Because of his history of PE and physical examination findings, a transthoracic echocardiogram was performed to evaluate for pulmonary hypertension. The echocardiogram demonstrated RV dilation and moderate tricuspid regurgitation (Fig. 11.1) with a severely

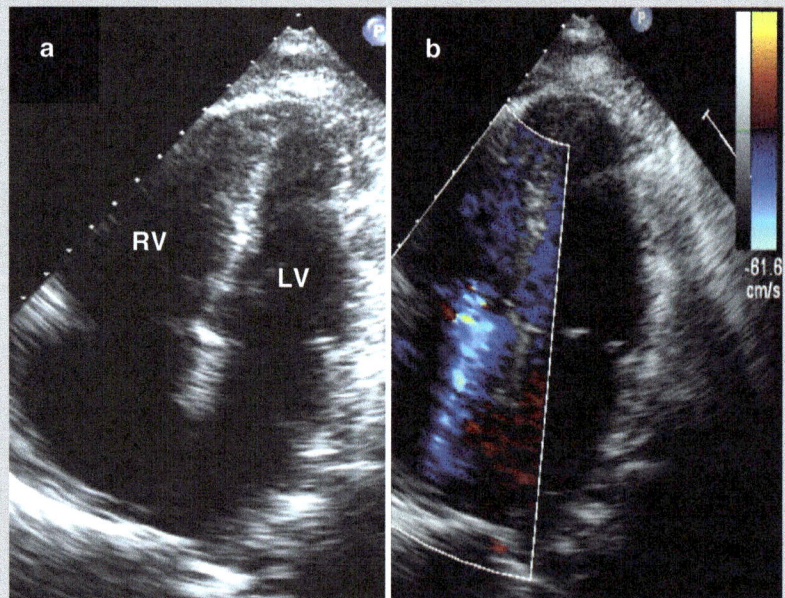

Fig. 11.1 Transthoracic echocardiogram, apical four-chamber view, demonstrating a dilated right ventricle (*RV*) compared with the left ventricle (*LV*) (**panel a**) in a 69-year-old man with prior pulmonary embolism (PE) and progressive dyspnea on exertion. Color Doppler echocardiography showed moderate tricuspid regurgitation (*blue color* jet) (**panel b**)

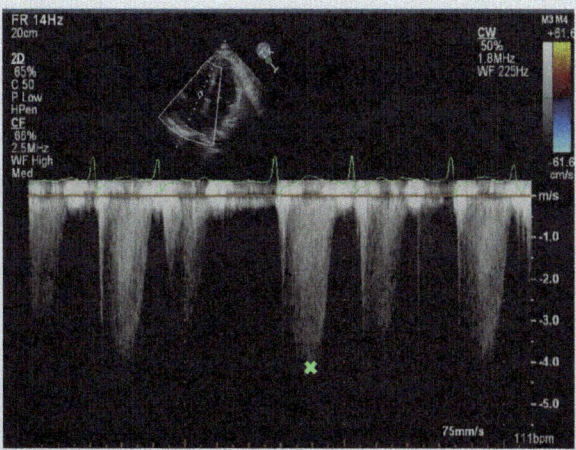

Fig. 11.2 Transthoracic echocardiogram, apical four-chamber view, demonstrating moderate pulmonary hypertension as defined by a peak tricuspid regurgitant jet velocity (X) of at least 400 cm/s in a 69-year-old man with prior pulmonary embolism (PE) and progressive dyspnea on exertion. Using the modified Bernoulli equation ($4\times$ [peak tricuspid regurgitant jet velocity]^2 + the estimate of right atrial pressure), the estimated pulmonary artery systolic pressure was 84 mmHg

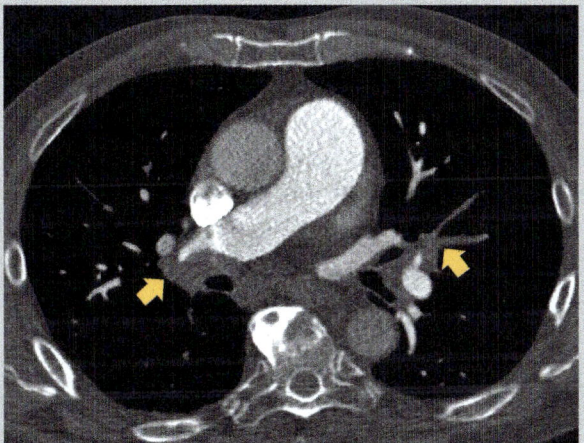

Fig. 11.3 Contrast-enhanced chest computed tomogram (CT) demonstrating extensive obstruction of right main pulmonary artery and branches of the left main pulmonary artery (*arrows*) with chronic thromboembolic material in a 69-year-old man with prior pulmonary embolism (PE), progressive dyspnea on exertion, and severe pulmonary hypertension

elevated estimated pulmonary artery systolic pressure of 84 mmHg (Fig. 11.2). A contrast-enhanced chest CT demonstrated extensive chronic bilateral PE consistent with chronic thromboembolic pulmonary hypertension (Fig. 11.3). After definitive therapy with surgical pulmonary thromboendarterectomy, the patient's exertional dyspnea completely resolved.

Epidemiology

Chronic thromboembolic pulmonary hypertension (CTEPH) may follow both single and recurrent episodes of PE (often asymptomatic) and is characterized by persistent macrovascular obstruction, pulmonary vasoconstriction, and a secondary small-vessel arteriopathy [1]. CTEPH used to be considered a rare complication but is now recognized to occur in 2–4 % of patients after PE. CTEPH is often overlooked because many patients lack a history of clinically overt PE. The risk of developing CTEPH is increased by PE-specific factors, certain chronic medical conditions, thrombophilia, and genetic predisposition (Table 11.1).

Pathophysiology

CTEPH results in persistent macrovascular obstruction and pulmonary vasoconstriction. Neurohumoral factors, including endothelin-1, play an integral role in CTEPH pathogenesis, both as potent vasoconstrictors as well as triggers of microvascular changes. Decreased cross-sectional area of the pulmonary arteries due to thrombosis and vasoconstriction prompts further abnormal vascular remodeling. In situ thrombosis may also accompany the secondary small-vessel arteriopathy. The secondary small vessel arteriopathy is characterized by medial hypertrophy, intimal proliferation, microvascular thrombosis, and plexiform lesion formation.

The combination of persistent macrovascular obstruction, secondary small vessel arteriopathy, and vasoconstriction results in pulmonary hypertension and right ventricular pressure overload that typically exceeds the level expected from PE-related pulmonary arterial obstruction alone.

Clinical Presentation

Exercise intolerance, fatigue, and dyspnea are the most commonly reported symptoms. As the disease progresses, patients may report chest discomfort, syncope, hemoptysis, lightheadedness, or peripheral leg edema. While patients may be initially asymptomatic, CTEPH often progresses to debilitating exercise intolerance, chronic dyspnea, and may result in chronic right ventricular (RV) failure. Diagnostic delays are common because many patients do not provide a history of PE. The patient in the Clinical Vignette suffered a delay in diagnosis because his persistent dyspnea was attributed to a slow recovery from his PE. Transthoracic echocardiography performed between 6 weeks after an acute PE has been suggested to screen for persistent pulmonary hypertension that may predict the development of CTEPH [2].

Table 11.1 Risk factors for chronic thromboembolic pulmonary hypertension (CTEPH)

Pulmonary embolism (PE)-specific factors
Recurrent or unprovoked PE
Larger lung scan perfusion defects at the time of PE presentation
Young or elderly age at the time of PE
Pulmonary artery systolic pressure >50 mmHg at initial PE presentation
Persistent pulmonary hypertension performed 6 months after acute PE
Chronic medical disorders
Infected surgical cardiac shunts or pacemaker/defibrillator leads
Splenectomy
Inflammatory diseases
Thyroid disease
Malignancy
Pro-thrombotic factors
Lupus anticoagulant or antiphospholipid antibodies
Increased factor VIII levels
Dysfibrinogenemia
Genetic factors
ABO blood groups other than O
Human leukocyte antigen (HLA) polymorphisms
Abnormal endogenous fibrinolysis

Physical examination findings are largely nonspecific and suggest the presence of pulmonary hypertension: reduction in the splitting of the second heart sound (S2), accentuation of the sound of pulmonic closure (P2), and a palpable right ventricular heave. Later findings correlate with declining RV function: jugular venous distension, fixed splitting of S2, a right-sided third heart sound (S3), tricuspid regurgitation, hepatomegaly, ascites, and peripheral edema.

Diagnosis

After a thorough history and physical examination, patients with symptoms and signs of pulmonary hypertension and a clinical history compatible with PE or pulmonary hypertension of unexplained etiology should be evaluated for CTEPH with imaging tests (Fig. 11.4). Echocardiography is sensitive for the detection of pulmonary hypertension and RV dysfunction but is not specific for the diagnosis of CTEPH. Ventilation perfusion (V/Q) lung scanning usually shows perfusion defects with normal ventilation, thus differentiating CTEPH from other causes of pulmonary hypertension but does not anatomically localize the extent of disease or determine surgical accessibility [3]. Contrast-enhanced chest CT may complement the

Fig. 11.4 Algorithm for the diagnosis of chronic thromboembolic pulmonary hypertension (*CTEPH*). *PE* pulmonary embolism, *CT* computed tomography

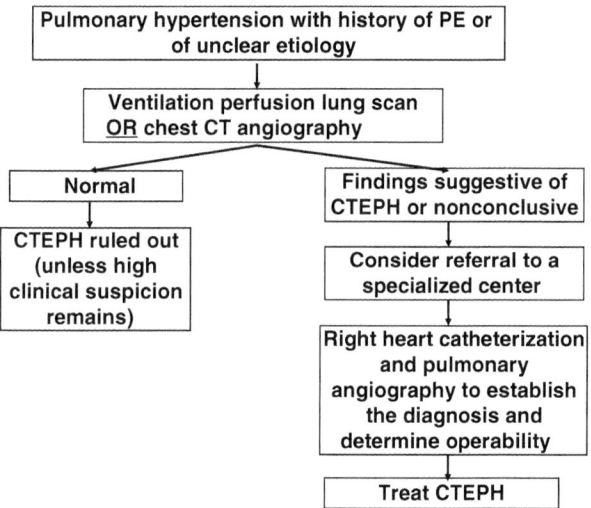

information obtained from ventilation-perfusion lung scanning by providing additional data, in particular anatomical localization and surgical accessibility.

If either chest CT or ventilation-perfusion lung scanning is inconclusive for CTEPH or if surgery is being considered, right heart catheterization and invasive pulmonary angiography will confirm the diagnosis and further define the anatomy. Right heart catheterization performed in conjunction with invasive pulmonary angiography quantifies the degree of pulmonary hypertension and can be used to assess responsiveness to vasodilator therapy. Patients with pulmonary hypertension and findings of PE on chest CT or ventilation-perfusion lung scanning should be referred to specialized centers and evaluated by multidisciplinary teams.

Treatment

Pulmonary Thromboendarterectomy

Pulmonary thromboendarterectomy is the most effective therapy for CTEPH. Patients with symptomatic CTEPH, surgically accessible disease, and an acceptable perioperative mortality should be referred for pulmonary thromboendarterectomy. Successful surgery removes obstructive chronic thromboembolic material and markedly improves the hemodynamic parameters of pulmonary artery pressure, pulmonary vascular resistance, and cardiac output (Fig. 11.5) [4, 5]. Symptoms and functional status improve accordingly, and improvements are typically sustained over time [5, 6]. Pulmonary thromboendarterectomy is performed under cardiopulmonary bypass with intermittent circulatory arrest to permit dissection from the main pulmonary arteries to the subsegmental branches. Inferior vena cava filters are often inserted perioperatively. The patient in the Clinical Vignette underwent pulmonary thromboendarterectomy at an experienced center with excellent results.

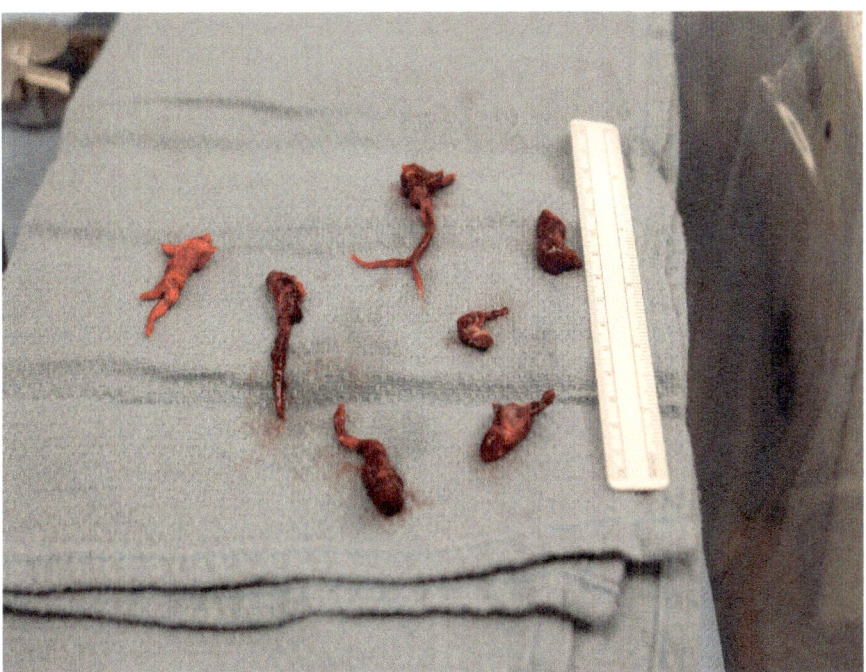

Fig. 11.5 Chronic thromboembolic material removed during pulmonary thromboendartectomy in a patient with history of recurrent pulmonary embolism (PE) and severe dyspnea on exertion who was found to have severe chronic thromboembolic pulmonary hypertension (Image courtesy of Dr. Ralph M Bolman, III)

Balloon Pulmonary Artery Angioplasty

Balloon pulmonary artery angioplasty is an option for selected patients who have inoperable disease due to distal surgically inaccessible disease or persistent or recurrent pulmonary hypertension after thromboendarterectomy. Balloon pulmonary artery angioplasty may reduce pulmonary artery pressure in patients with CTEPH [7]. Improvement in New York Heart Association functional class and 6-min walk capacity has also been observed after successful balloon pulmonary artery angioplasty. Experience with balloon pulmonary artery angioplasty is very limited, and the procedure should be performed at experienced centers.

Medical Therapy

Anticoagulation

Anticoagulation is prescribed in the majority of patients with CTEPH, although randomized clinical trial data are lacking. The rationale for anticoagulation is to prevent in situ pulmonary artery thrombosis and recurrent venous thromboembolism (VTE).

In patients who had unprovoked (idiopathic) PE, numerous studies show that indefinite duration anticoagulation reduces the risk of recurrent VTE [8, 9].

Pulmonary Vasodilators

Up to 50 % of patients with CTEPH are inoperable and 10 % of post-thromboendarterectomy patients suffer persistent or recurrent pulmonary hypertension. Patients with CTEPH show acute vasoreactivity to inhaled pulmonary vasodilators, suggesting at least some degree of shared pathophysiology [10]. Pulmonary vasodilators offer these patients the promise of improved symptoms and functional capacity. Advanced medical therapies include the endothelin receptor antagonist, bosentan [11], the phosphodiesterase inhibitor, sildenafil [12], a novel guanylate cyclase stimulator, riociguat [13], and prostacyclin analogues, such as epoprostenol or treprostinil. Combination therapy titrated to the patients' symptoms and functional status is an emerging option.

Overall Therapeutic Algorithm

The key decision point in CTEPH therapy is to identify patients with surgically accessible chronic thromboembolic disease in whom pulmonary thromboendarterectomy will likely result in a substantial reduction in pulmonary vascular resistance (Fig. 11.6). Vasodilators should be reserved for patients with inoperable disease or those with persistent or recurrent CTEPH after pulmonary thromboendarterectomy. Patients with CTEPH in whom pulmonary thromboendarterectomy or vasodilator therapy is contemplated should be referred to specialized centers with experience in the management of CTEPH and where dedicated treatment protocols and enrollment in clinical trials may be offered.

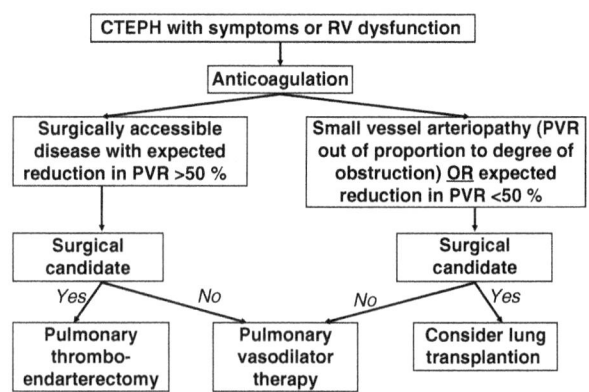

Fig. 11.6 Algorithm for management of chronic thromboembolic pulmonary hypertension (*CTEPH*). *RV* right ventricular, *PVR* pulmonary vascular resistance

Answer Key

1. **Correct answer**, (**d**) Systemic fibrinolytic therapy is not a risk factor for CTEPH. In fact, systemic fibrinolysis may actually prevent CTEPH.
2. **Correct answer**, (**c**) Surgical pulmonary thromboendarterectomy is the most effective therapy for CTEPH. Successful surgery removes obstructive chronic thromboembolic material and improves pulmonary hypertension, pulmonary vascular resistance, and cardiac output. Surgery results in durable improvements in symptoms and functional status.

References

1. Piazza G, Goldhaber SZ. Chronic thromboembolic pulmonary hypertension. N Engl J Med. 2011;364:351–60.
2. Jaff MR, McMurtry MS, Archer SL, et al. Management of massive and submassive pulmonary embolism, iliofemoral deep vein thrombosis, and chronic thromboembolic pulmonary hypertension: a scientific statement from the American Heart Association. Circulation. 2011;123: 1788–830.
3. Tunariu N, Gibbs SJ, Win Z, et al. Ventilation-perfusion scintigraphy is more sensitive than multidetector CTPA in detecting chronic thromboembolic pulmonary disease as a treatable cause of pulmonary hypertension. J Nucl Med. 2007;48:680–4.
4. Piovella F, D'Armini AM, Barone M, Tapson VF. Chronic thromboembolic pulmonary hypertension. Semin Thromb Hemost. 2006;32:848–55.
5. Corsico AG, D'Armini AM, Cerveri I, et al. Long-term outcome after pulmonary endarterectomy. Am J Respir Crit Care Med. 2008;178:419–24.
6. Matsuda H, Ogino H, Minatoya K, et al. Long-term recovery of exercise ability after pulmonary endarterectomy for chronic thromboembolic pulmonary hypertension. Ann Thorac Surg. 2006;82:1338–43.
7. Feinstein JA, Goldhaber SZ, Lock JE, Ferndandes SM, Landzberg MJ. Balloon pulmonary angioplasty for treatment of chronic thromboembolic pulmonary hypertension. Circulation. 2001;103:10–3.
8. Goldhaber SZ, Piazza G. Optimal duration of anticoagulation after venous thromboembolism. Circulation. 2011;123:664–7.
9. Kearon C, Akl EA, Comerota AJ, et al. Antithrombotic therapy for VTE disease: antithrombotic therapy and prevention of thrombosis, 9th ed: American College of Chest Physicians Evidence-Based Clinical Practice Guidelines. Chest. 2012;141:e419S–94.
10. Ulrich S, Fischler M, Speich R, Popov V, Maggiorini M. Chronic thromboembolic and pulmonary arterial hypertension share acute vasoreactivity properties. Chest. 2006;130:841–6.
11. Jais X, D'Armini AM, Jansa P, et al. Bosentan for treatment of inoperable chronic thromboembolic pulmonary hypertension: BENEFiT (Bosentan Effects in iNopErable Forms of chronIc Thromboembolic pulmonary hypertension), a randomized, placebo-controlled trial. J Am Coll Cardiol. 2008;52:2127–34.
12. Ghofrani HA, Schermuly RT, Rose F, et al. Sildenafil for long-term treatment of nonoperable chronic thromboembolic pulmonary hypertension. Am J Respir Crit Care Med. 2003;167: 1139–41.
13. Ghofrani HA, D'Armini AM, Grimminger F, et al. Riociguat for the treatment of chronic thromboembolic pulmonary hypertension. N Engl J Med. 2013;369:319–29.

Chapter 12
Post-thrombotic Syndrome: Recognizing and Treating a Debilitating Complication of Deep Vein Thrombosis

Abstract Post-thrombotic syndrome (PTS) is a debilitating long-term complication of deep vein thrombosis (DVT). Patients with PTS present with chronic lower extremity edema, hyperpigmentation, and, in advanced cases, venous ulceration. PTS results in substantial disability, loss of functional status, and health care expenditure. Compression therapy, including graduated compression stockings, comprises the cornerstone of PTS therapy.

Keywords Chronic venous insufficiency • Deep vein thrombosis • Diagnosis • Post-thrombotic syndrome • Treatment

Self-Assessment Questions

1. Which of the following physical examination findings is not indicative of post-thrombotic syndrome (PTS) in a patient with prior deep vein thrombosis (DVT)?

   (a) Varicose veins
   (b) Pitting edema
   (c) Atrophie blanche
   (d) Erythema nodosum

2. Which of the following is the cornerstone of therapy for PTS?

   (a) Angioplasty and venous stenting
   (b) Graduated compression stockings
   (c) Horse chestnut seed extract
   (d) Surgical venous bypass

© Springer International Publishing Switzerland 2015   111
G. Piazza et al., *Handbook for Venous Thromboembolism*,
DOI 10.1007/978-3-319-20843-5_12

Clinical Vignette

A 77-year-old woman was admitted to a regional hospital Trauma Intensive Care Unit (ICU) following a high-speed motor vehicle accident with multiple injuries, including bilateral pelvic fractures, left-sided rib fractures, left pneumothorax, a right orbital fracture, and a concussion. Her prolonged hospital course was complicated by bilateral common femoral DVTs despite compression stockings and prophylactic dose subcutaneous unfractionated heparin. She was initiated on intravenous unfractionated heparin as a "bridge" to oral anticoagulation with warfarin. She was eventually discharged home with a plan for 6 months of anticoagulation with warfarin. At her 6 month follow-up visit with her Primary Care Physician, she continued to complain of lower extremity edema, "heaviness," and "brownish-red discoloration" of her legs around the ankles. On physical examination, she had 2+ pitting edema bilaterally, brown hyperpigmentation above the right medial malleolus, and a reddish hue to her lower legs (Fig. 12.1). Her Primary Care Physician ordered bilateral venous ultrasounds to evaluate for new or residual DVT. Venous ultrasounds demonstrated partial non-compressibility of the bilateral common femoral veins (Fig. 12.2) and small channels of

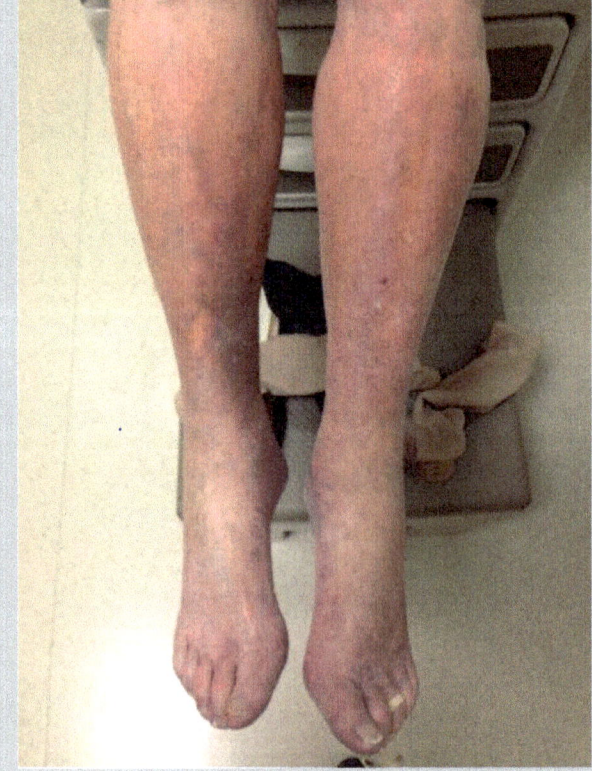

Fig. 12.1 Physical examination demonstrating bilateral lower extremity edema and reddish discoloration with hyperpigmentation above the right medial malleolus consistent with post-thrombotic syndrome (PTS) in a 77-year-old woman with bilateral deep vein thrombosis (DVT) diagnosed 6 months prior following a motor vehicle accident

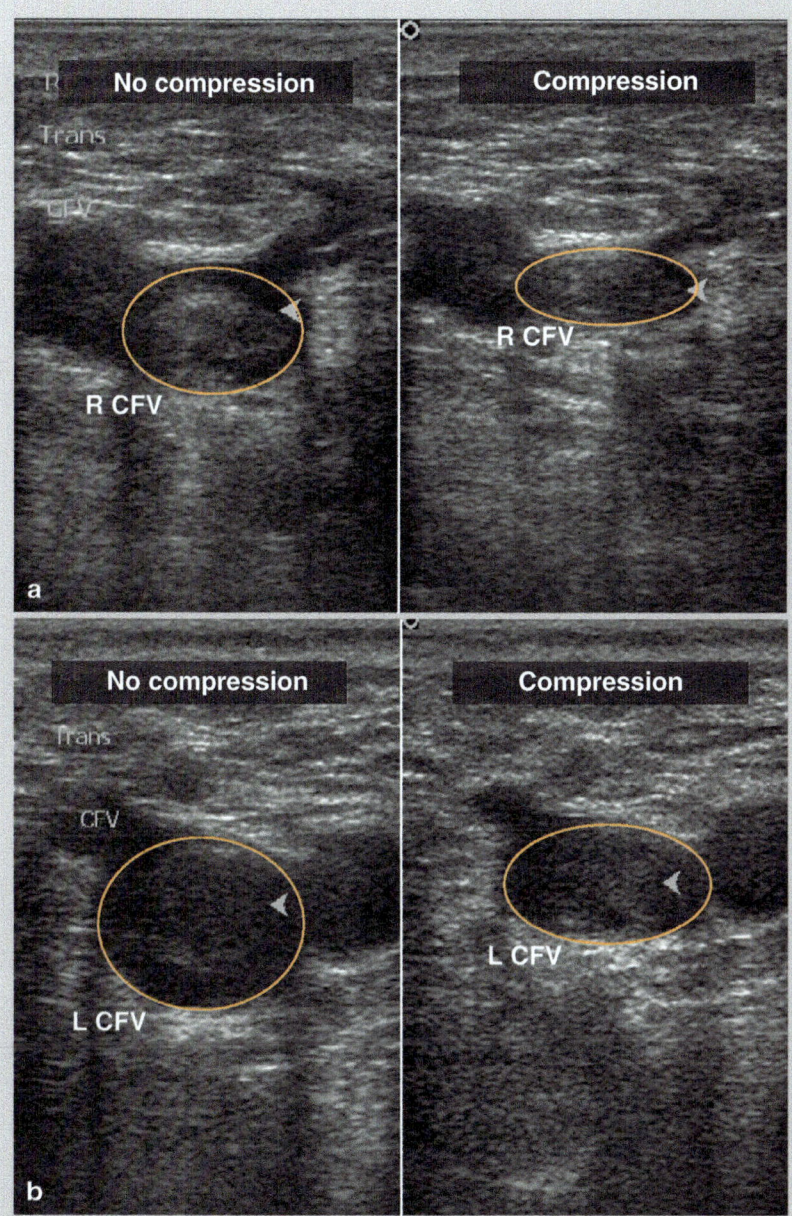

Fig. 12.2 Venous ultrasound demonstrating partial non-compressibility (*ovals*) of the bilateral common femoral veins (*R CFV* and *L CFV*) consistent with chronic-appearing deep vein thrombosis (DVT) in a 77-year-old woman with bilateral DVT diagnosed 6 months prior following a motor vehicle accident and ongoing symptoms of edema and lower extremity discomfort (**Panel a** and **b**). The DVT is represented by the hyperechoic material (*arrowheads*) in the lumen of the common femoral veins (**Panel a** and **b**)

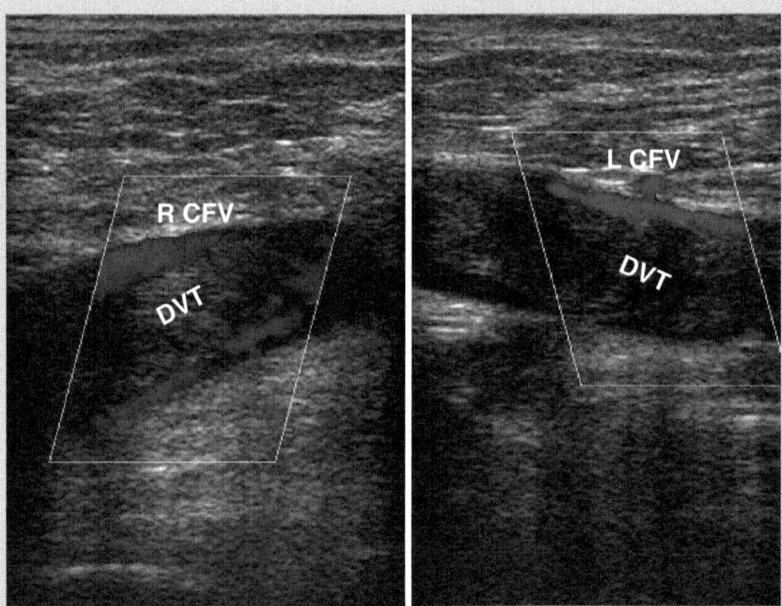

Fig. 12.3 Venous ultrasound demonstrating small channels of color Doppler flow (*blue*) consistent with partially recanalized chronic-appearing deep vein thrombosis (*DVT*) in the bilateral common femoral veins (*R CFV* and *L CFV*) of a 77-year-old woman with bilateral DVT diagnosed 6 months prior following a motor vehicle accident and ongoing symptoms of edema and lower extremity discomfort

color Doppler flow consistent with partially recanalized chronic-appearing DVT (Fig. 12.3). She was continued on anticoagulation with warfarin and referred to Vascular Medicine clinic for further evaluation. The Vascular Medicine provider diagnosed her with post-thrombotic syndrome (PTS) on the basis of her persistent symptoms despite 6 months of therapeutic antico-agulation for DVT. She was prescribed thigh high, 30–40 mmHg, graduated compression stockings to be used daily. Over the course of the next few months, the patient noted a marked improvement in her lower extremity edema and discomfort.

Post-thrombotic syndrome (PTS) is a common and debilitating long-term complica-tion of deep vein thrombosis (DVT). Depending on particular study, the frequency of PTS in patients treated with anticoagulation for acute DVT ranges from 25 to 50 % [1]. Patient-centered outcomes, including physical and mental well-being, quality of life, and symptom severity, as measured by the Short Form 36 (SF-36) Health Survey and the Venous Insufficiency Epidemiological and Economic Study (VEINES) questionnaire demonstrate lower scores (poorer outcomes) in patients

Table 12.1 Risk factors for post-thrombotic syndrome (PTS)

Incomplete resolution of deep vein thrombosis (DVT) symptoms by 1 month of anticoagulation
Iliofemoral DVT
Recurrent ipsilateral DVT
Increased body mass index (BMI)
Advanced age
Subtherapeutic anticoagulation > 50 % of the time during the first 3 months of therapy after DVT diagnosis

with PTS compared with those without [2]. PTS causes significant patient disability, loss of functional status, lost days at work, and substantial health care expenditures, especially if venous ulcerations form. Failure to recognize PTS can result in excessive courses of therapeutic anticoagulation as well as unnecessary and costly serial venous ultrasounds.

Pathophysiology

Risk factors for PTS include iliofemoral DVT, recurrent ipsilateral DVT, incomplete resolution of DVT symptoms after 1 month of therapeutic anticoagulation, increasing body mass index (BMI), advanced age, and suboptimal anticoagulation during the first 3 months after DVT diagnosis (Table 12.1). The patient in the Clinical Vignette suffered bilateral DVT at the junction of the external iliac and common femoral veins, placing her at increased risk for PTS. The pathophysiology of PTS involves persistent venous outflow obstruction and venous valvular damage and incompetence, resulting in venous hypertension [3]. An inflammatory response to DVT in the wall of the vein causes further venous valvular injury and dysfunction. The combination of local inflammation and venous hypertension leads to capillary leak and clinical findings of edema, hyperpigmentation, and eventual ulceration.

Although PTS typically occurs as a complication of lower extremity DVT, it can also develop following upper extremity DVT.

Clinical Presentation

Symptoms of PTS include lower extremity discomfort (in particular "heaviness" and pain), leg fatigue, and swelling. The clinical presentation comprises a spectrum of physical examination findings of chronic venous insufficiency ranging from venous ectasia, such as spider, reticular, and varicose veins, edema, hyperpigmentation, lipodermatosclerosis, atrophie blanche, and venous ulceration

Fig. 12.4 Physical examination demonstrating severe edema and hyperpigmentation consistent with post-thrombotic syndrome (PTS) in a 37-year-old man with history of prior recurrent left lower extremity deep vein thromboisis (DVT)

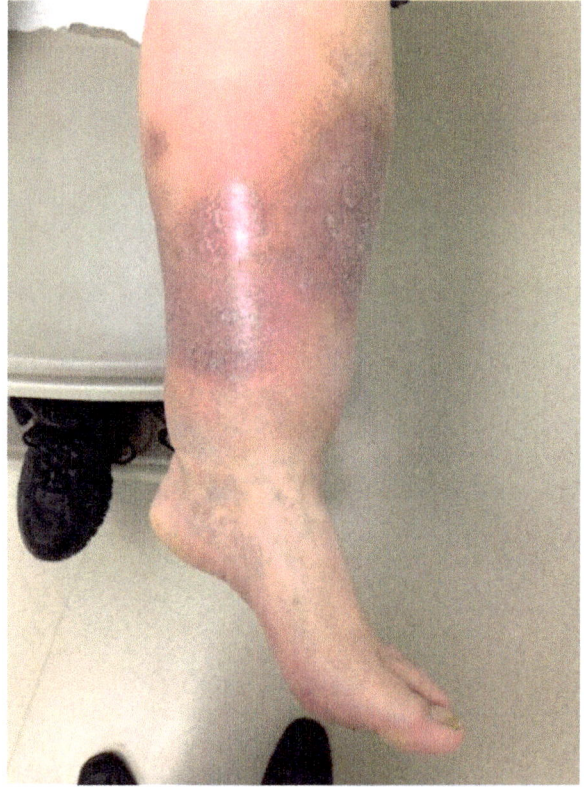

(Figs. 12.4, 12.5, and 12.6) [4]. Although the areas around the medial malleoli are the typical locations for PTS, findings of venous ectasia, hyperpigmentation, and ulceration can be observed elsewhere in the lower extremity. Patients with PTS are prone to recurrent lower extremity cellulitis (Fig. 12.7).

PTS must be distinguished from other causes of lower extremity edema (Table 12.2)

Diagnosis

PTS is a clinical diagnosis and does not require any laboratory testing or imaging. The diagnosis of PTS is made when patients have a history of prior DVT and 3–6 months from the initial diagnosis have persistent symptoms, signs of chronic venous insufficiency, or both. Venous ultrasound, if performed, may demonstrate chronic DVT or deep venous reflux.

Fig. 12.5 Physical examination demonstrating a patchy loss of pigmentation around the right medial malleolus, known as atrophie blanche, in a 66-year-old woman with prior deep vein thrombosis (DVT) after right knee arthroplasty who developed post-thrombotic syndrome (PTS)

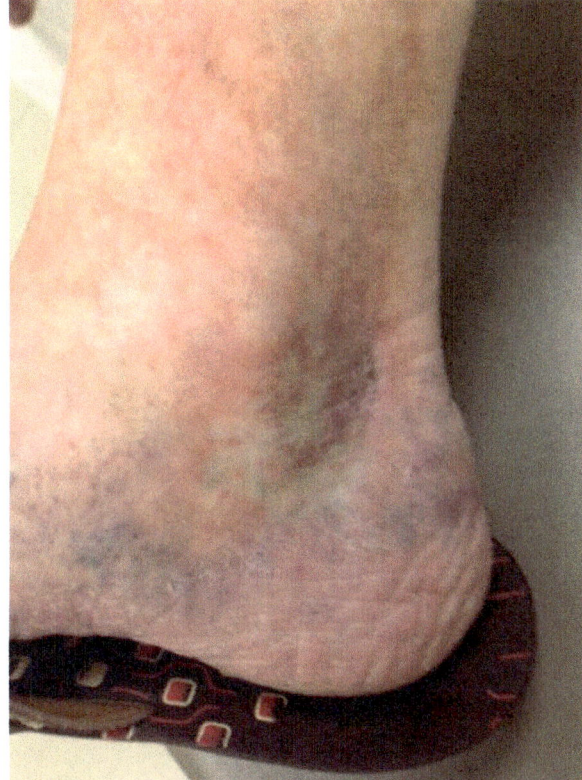

Treatment

Compression therapy is the cornerstone of therapy for PTS [1]. Compression therapy helps to alleviate patient's symptoms of lower extremity discomfort and swelling and prevent venous ulceration [5, 6]. Patients with PTS should be prescribed graduated compression stockings, with a minimum strength of 30–40 mmHg and a length sufficient to cover the symptomatic areas of the limb. The patient in the Clinical Vignette demonstrated an excellent response to graduate compression stocking therapy. The stocking prescription should be renewed every 3 months, because the stockings lose their elasticity, especially if laundered frequently.

Compression wraps and short-stretch bandages may be helpful in patients with PTS and limbs that are too edematous to fit into standard compression stockings. Home pneumatic compression pumps may also help reduce symptoms [7]. Frequent elevation (at least 30 min, four times per day) can also help with limb decongestion. Exercise training may also improve PTS symptoms [8].

Fig. 12.6 Physical examination demonstrating healed recurrent venous ulcerations above the lateral malleolus in a 69-year-old woman with long-standing post-thrombotic syndrome (PTS) many years after suffering extensive left deep vein thrombosis (DVT) in the setting of pregnancy

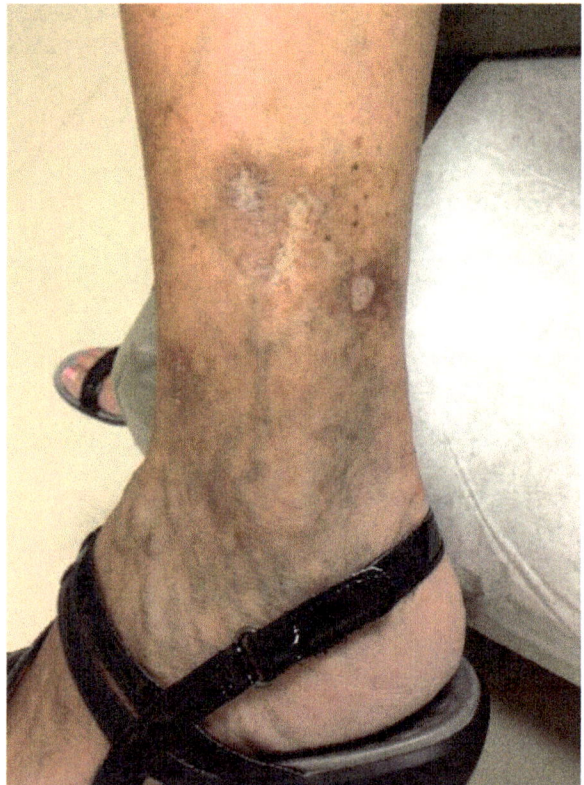

For patients with open venous ulcerations, zinc paste bandages can be used. Management of venous ulcerations is best accomplished through a wound care clinic. Venous ulcerations should always be examined for superimposed infection.

Options for pharmacological therapy for PTS are limited. In patients with chronic venous insufficiency, horse chestnut seed extract, a venoactive drug, has been shown to improve symptoms and reduce lower extremity volume and circumference [9]. The efficacy of horse chestnut seed extract in patients with PTS remains unproven.

Varicose veins in patients with PTS are best treated with compression therapy. Ablative therapies for varicose veins, such as surgical vein stripping or endovenous radiofrequency or laser ablation, may worsen lower extremity symptoms in patients with PTS because removal or closure of the superficial venous system runs the risk of forcing more venous return via the obstructed deep venous system.

Percutaneous venous intervention may be considered for patients with PTS and chronic caval or iliac venous stenosis or occlusion. Angioplasty with or without venous stenting has a high technical success rate (95 %) at experienced centers and improves venous clinical severity scores [10]. Surgical venous bypass and venous valve reconstruction may be considered when endovascular therapies have failed and are limited to a select few high-volume centers.

Fig. 12.7 Physical examination demonstrating severe edema and hyperpigmentation above the medial malleolus with erythema, warmth, and tenderness in a 58-year-old man with prior left lower extremity DVT, findings of post-thrombotic syndrome (PTS), and superimposed cellulitis

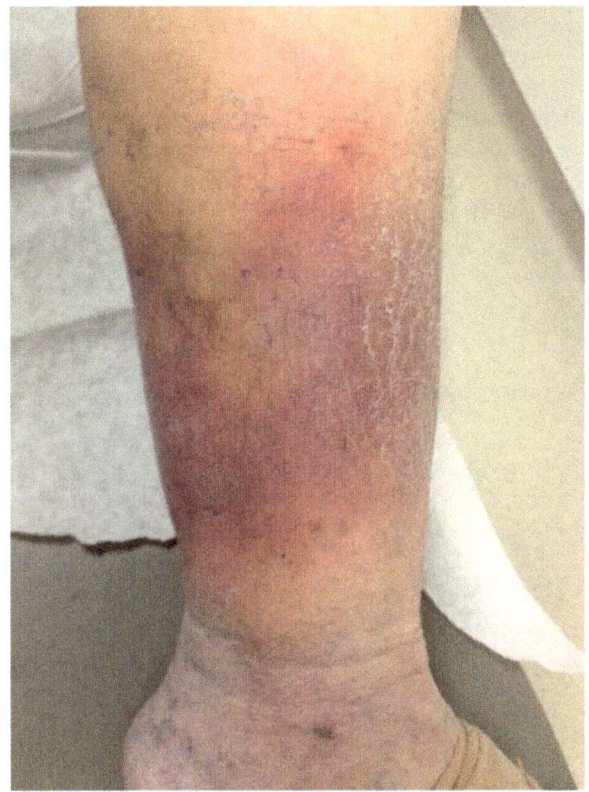

Table 12.2 Differential diagnosis of lower extremity edema

Local causes	Systemic causes
Deep vein thrombosis	Thyroid disease
Lymphedema	Renal disease
Chronic venous insufficiency	Liver disease
	Medications
May-Thurner syndrome	Left heart failure
Lipedema	Right heart failure
Venous compression syndromes	Salt retention
Venous stenosis	Hypoalbuminemia
Cellulitis	Idiopathic
Allergic reactions	

Prevention

Although common practice, prescription of graduated compression stockings following diagnosis of acute DVT has not been proven to prevent post-thrombotic syndrome [11]. Catheter-assisted thrombectomy ("pharmacomechanical therapy") in patients with iliofemoral or femoral DVT may help to prevent PTS. In the

European CaVenT study, 209 patients with first-time iliofemoral DVT were randomized to standard anticoagulation alone or in combination with catheter-directed fibrinolysis [12]. At 24 months, the rate of post-thrombotic syndrome was reduced in patients who underwent pharmacomechanical therapy compared with those assigned to standard anticoagulation alone (41.1 % vs. 55.6 %, p=0.047). The National Heart Lung and Blood Institute (NHLBI)-sponsored ATTRACT Trial (ClinicalTrials.gov Identifier: NCT00790335) has completed enrollment and will determine if pharmacomechanical therapy can safely prevent post-thrombotic syndrome.

Answer Key

1. **Correct answer**, (**d**) Varicose veins, pitting edema, and atrophie blanche are all findings of PTS. Erythema nodosum is associated with certain infections, chronic inflammatory disorders, medications, pregnancy, and malignancy but not PTS.
2. **Correct answer**, (**b**) Compression therapy is the cornerstone of therapy for PTS. Compression therapy helps to alleviate patient's symptoms of lower extremity discomfort and swelling and prevent venous ulceration. The other therapies may be considered when compression therapy fails to improve symptoms.

References

1. Kahn SR, Comerota AJ, Cushman M, et al. The postthrombotic syndrome: evidence-based prevention, diagnosis, and treatment strategies: a scientific statement from the American Heart Association. Circulation. 2014;130:1636–61.
2. Kahn SR, Shbaklo H, Lamping DL, et al. Determinants of health-related quality of life during the 2 years following deep vein thrombosis. J Thromb Haemost. 2008;6:1105–12.
3. Kahn SR. How I treat postthrombotic syndrome. Blood. 2009;114:4624–31.
4. Kahn SR, Shrier I, Julian JA, et al. Determinants and time course of the postthrombotic syndrome after acute deep venous thrombosis. Ann Intern Med. 2008;149:698–707.
5. Cohen JM, Akl EA, Kahn SR. Pharmacologic and compression therapies for postthrombotic syndrome: a systematic review of randomized controlled trials. Chest. 2012;141:308–20.
6. Lattimer CR, Azzam M, Kalodiki E, Makris GC, Geroulakos G. Compression stockings significantly improve hemodynamic performance in post-thrombotic syndrome irrespective of class or length. J Vasc Surg. 2013;58:158–65.
7. Levi M. A long-awaited small step forward in the management of the post-thrombotic syndrome. Thromb Haemost. 2008;99:463–4.
8. Kahn SR, Shrier I, Shapiro S, et al. Six-month exercise training program to treat postthrombotic syndrome: a randomized controlled two-centre trial. CMAJ. 2011;183:37–44.
9. Pittler MH, Ernst E. Horse chestnut seed extract for chronic venous insufficiency. Cochrane Database Syst Rev. 2012;(11):CD003230.

10. Hartung O, Otero A, Boufi M, et al. Mid-term results of endovascular treatment for symptomatic chronic nonmalignant iliocaval venous occlusive disease. J Vasc Surg. 2005;42:1138–44; discussion 1144.
11. Kahn SR, Shapiro S, Wells PS, et al. Compression stockings to prevent post-thrombotic syndrome: a randomised placebo-controlled trial. Lancet. 2014;383:880–8.
12. Enden T, Haig Y, Klow NE, et al. Long-term outcome after additional catheter-directed thrombolysis versus standard treatment for acute iliofemoral deep vein thrombosis (the CaVenT study): a randomised controlled trial. Lancet. 2012;379:31–8.

Chapter 13
Prevention of Venous Thromboembolism: An Evidence-Based Approach to Thromboprophylaxis

Abstract Although evidence-based practice guidelines for prevention of venous thromboembolism (VTE) among hospitalized patients have been published, implementation of thromboprophylaxis continues to be inconsistent in the U.S., Canada, and worldwide. Quality Improvement initiatives, including decision support-based strategies, have the potential to improve prophylaxis utilization and reduce the incidence of VTE during hospitalization. The approach to VTE prevention among hospitalized and postoperative patients must consider the patient population and individual risk while integrating the use of mechanical and pharmacological modalities when indicated.

Keywords Mechanical prophylaxis • Pharmacological prophylaxis • Prevention • Thromboprophylaxis

Self-Assessment Questions

1. Which of the following has not been shown to prevent VTE in high-risk hospitalized patients?

    (a) Enoxaparin 40 mg subcutaneously daily
    (b) Fondaparinux 2.5 mg subcutaneously daily
    (c) 4-factor prothrombin complex concentrate (PCC) 50 U/kg intravenously daily
    (d) An electronic alert notifying providers that the patient is at increased risk for VTE and is not ordered for any prophylactic measures

2. Which of the following is the most critical initial step for ensuring appropriate VTE preventive measures in hospitalized Medical Service patients?

    (a) Quality Improvement initiatives to encourage pharmacological prophylaxis in all Medical Service patients
    (b) VTE and bleeding risk assessment in all Medical Service patients prior to initiation of VTE prophylaxis

(c) Default "opt-out" orders for graduated compression stockings for all Medical Service patients upon admission

(d) A patient-level education program focused on VTE risk and prevention for all Medical Service inpatients

Clinical Vignette

A 44-year-old obese woman admitted to the Medical Service with pyelonephritis had been improving on parenteral antibiotics when she developed chest pain and dyspnea. The "Nightfloat" Medicine Resident evaluated the patient urgently. On physical examination, the patient was tachycardic to 120 beats per minute, normotensive with a blood pressure of 136/74 mmHg, tachypneic to 24 breaths per minute, and hypoxemic to 94 % on 6 L oxygen by nasal cannula. Pneumatic compression boots and graduated compression stockings were noted on the floor by the foot of the hospital bed. An electrocardiogram was remarkable for sinus tachycardia. A portable chest X-ray was unremarkable. Because of concern for pulmonary embolism (PE), a contrast-enhanced chest computed tomogram (CT) was performed. The chest CT demonstrated a large "saddle" PE (Fig. 13.1) without any signs of right ventricular (RV) enlargement. The patient was immediately administered unfractionated heparin as an intravenous bolus followed by a continuous infusion. Upon

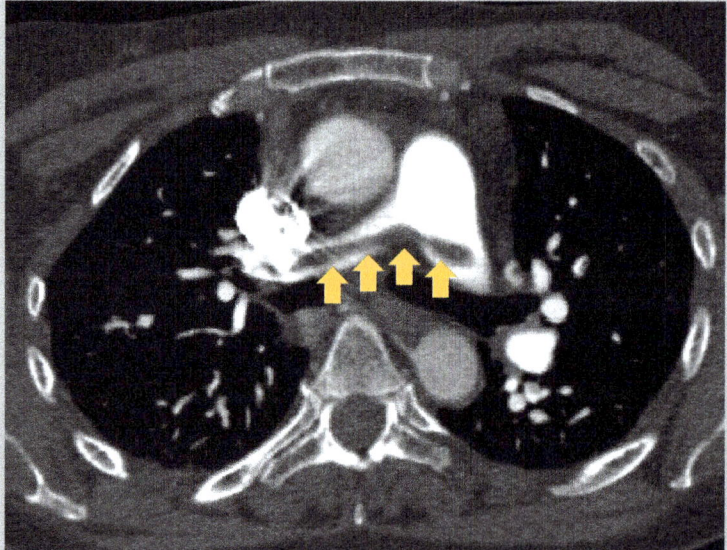

Fig. 13.1 Contrast-enhanced chest computed tomogram (CT) demonstrating large "saddle" pulmonary embolism (PE) (*arrows*) in a 44-year-old obese woman admitted with pyelonephritis and had been refusing pharmacological prophylaxis

review of the patient's medical record, the Medicine Resident noted that the patient had been prescribed prophylactic-dose enoxaparin. Per the nursing records, the patient had refused her enoxaparin injections for the prior 3 days.

The U.S. Surgeon General's 2008 Call To Action To Prevent Deep Vein Thrombosis and Pulmonary Embolism identified PE as the most preventable cause of death among hospitalized patients [1]. Although evidence-based practice guidelines for prevention of VTE among hospitalized patients have been published [2–4], implementation of thromboprophylaxis continues to be inconsistent in the U.S. [5], Canada [6], and worldwide [7, 8]. Quality Improvement initiatives, including decision support-based strategies, have the potential to improve thromboprophylaxis utilization and reduce the incidence of VTE during hospitalization [9–13]. The patient in the Clinical Vignette highlights the critical importance of Quality Improvement initiatives to prevent VTE in hospitalized patients, including patient education to improve adherence.

Options for Thromboprophylaxis

Mechanical Prophylaxis

Mechanical prophylactic modalities such as graduated compression stockings and intermittent pneumatic compression devices increase venous blood flow and may augment endogenous fibrinolysis, thereby leading to reductions in VTE [14]. Mechanical prophylaxis is frequently prescribed in patients at risk for VTE and who have contraindications to pharmacological prophylaxis. Mechanical VTE prophylaxis has been evaluated most recently in three trials of acute stroke patients.

In an outcome-blinded, randomized controlled trial, 2518 immobilized patients admitted to hospital within 1 week of an acute stroke were assigned to routine care plus thigh-length graduated compression stockings or to routine care alone [15]. The primary outcome of symptomatic or asymptomatic DVT in the popliteal or femoral veins occurred in 10 % patients randomized to thigh-length graduated compression stockings and 10.5 % assigned to the control group. Skin breakdown, ulceration, blisters, and skin necrosis were significantly more common in patients randomized to graduated compression stockings than in the control group (5 % vs. 1 %; odds ratio [OR] 4.18, 95 % confidence interval [CI] 2.40–7.27).

In a subsequent randomized controlled trial, 3114 immobile patients hospitalized with acute stroke were assigned to receive thigh-length graduated compression stockings or below-knee graduated compression stockings [16]. The primary outcome of symptomatic or asymptomatic DVT in the popliteal or femoral veins occurred in 6.3 % of patients who received thigh-length graduated compression stockings and 8.8 % of those who received below-knee graduated compression stockings (absolute difference, 2.5 %; 95 % CI, 0.7–4.4 %; p = 0.008). Skin breakdown occurred in 3.9 % of patients who received thigh-length graduated compression stockings and in 2.9 % of those who received below-knee graduated compression stockings.

A multicenter, randomized trial assessed pneumatic compression devices for VTE prevention in 2876 immobilized patients with acute stroke [17]. The primary outcome, DVT in the proximal veins detected on a screening venous ultrasound or any symptomatic objectively-confirmed DVT in the proximal veins within 30 days of randomization, occurred in 8.5 % of patients prescribed pneumatic compression devices and 12.1 % of those allocated to no pneumatic compression devices (absolute risk reduction, 3.6 %; 95 % CI 1.4–5.8). Excluding 323 patients who died before any primary outcome and 41 without any screening venous ultrasound, the adjusted OR was 0.65 (95 % CI 0.51–0.84; p = 0.001) in favor of pneumatic compression devices.

Because the safety and efficacy of graduated compression stockings for mechanical VTE prophylaxis remain unclear, some evidence-based guidelines recommend against their use and emphasize the importance of pharmacological prophylaxis [18]. Unfortunately, as was the case with the patient in the Clinical Vignette, adherence to mechanical prophylactic measures is often poor.

Pharmacologic Prophylaxis

Pharmacologic agents for the prevention of VTE include subcutaneously administered unfractionated heparin, LMWH, warfarin, and fondaparinux. Low dose aspirin is also effective for prevention of VTE in patients who have undergone total hip or total knee arthroplasty [19]. Evidence-based practice guidelines provide specific recommendations for pharmacological VTE prophylaxis in a variety of patient populations [2–4, 18, 20]. Novel oral anticoagulants, including dabigatran [21], rivaroxaban [22–24], apixaban [25–27], and edoxaban [28] have been evaluated for VTE prophylaxis in large randomized controlled trials. A second-generation antisense oligonucleotide that specifically reduces factor XI levels has been evaluated for prevention of VTE in patients undergoing total knee arthroplasty [29].

Optimal Duration of Prophylaxis

The risk of VTE persists after hospital discharge with a significant number of patients, especially those who are postoperative, experiencing DVT or PE while at rehabilitation centers, skilled nursing facilities, or even at home. Several studies have validated the use of extended VTE prophylaxis for up to 4–6 weeks in high-risk patient populations such as those undergoing extensive oncologic or major orthopedic surgery [30–32]. Randomized controlled trials of extended duration VTE prophylaxis after hospital discharge in hospitalized Medical Service patients have not demonstrated a net clinical benefit but suggest a trend toward it [22, 25, 33]. Accordingly, the 2012 American College of Chest Physicians (ACCP) Evidence-Based Clinical Practice Guidelines for Prevention of Venous Thromboembolism in Nonsurgical Patients suggests against extended duration VTE prophylaxis beyond the acute hospital stay in acutely ill medical patients [4].

Recommendations for Specific Patient Populations

Medical Inpatients

The American College of Physicians (ACP) recommends assessment of risk for VTE and bleeding in all medical patients prior to initiation of VTE prophylaxis [18]. The ACP recommends pharmacological VTE prophylaxis with heparin or a related drug for VTE in medical patients, unless the bleeding risk outweighs the anticipated benefits. Furthermore, the ACP recommends against the use of mechanical prophylaxis with graduated compression stockings for VTE prevention in medical patients.

Although pharmacological thromboprophylaxis is effective for prevention of VTE [34, 35], it does not improve survival among hospitalized Medical Service patients. A double-blind, placebo-controlled, randomized trial assessed the effect of subcutaneous enoxaparin (40 mg daily) versus placebo for 10–14 days in 8307 patients who were wearing graduated compression stockings on the rate of death from any cause among hospitalized, acutely ill medical patients [36]. Study inclusion required an age of at least 40 years and hospitalization for acute decompensated heart failure, severe systemic infection with at least one VTE risk factor, or active cancer. The rate of death from any cause at day 30 was 4.9 % in the enoxaparin group versus 4.8 % in the placebo group (risk ratio, 1.0; 95 % CI, 0.8–1.2; $p=0.83$). The rate of major bleeding was 0.4 % in the enoxaparin group and 0.3 % in the placebo group (risk ratio, 1.4; 95 % CI, 0.7–3.1; $p=0.35$). Based on these data, use of enoxaparin plus graduated compression stockings compared with graduated compression stockings alone did not reduce the rate of death from any cause among hospitalized, acutely ill medical patients.

Medical Patients After Discharge

Several randomized control trials evaluating the safety and efficacy of VTE prophylaxis in medical patients after discharge have been reported. In one of the initial studies of thromboprophylaxis in Medical Service patients after discharge,

Extended Clinical prophylaxis in Acutely Ill Medical patients (EXCLAIM), extended-duration enoxaparin 40 mg daily reduced VTE incidence compared with placebo (2.5 % vs. 4 %; absolute risk difference favoring enoxaparin, −1.53 % [95 % CI, −2.54 to −0.52 %]) but increased major bleeding (0.8 % vs. 0.3 %; absolute risk difference favoring placebo, 0.51 % [95 % CI, 0.12–0.89 %]) [33]. The Multicenter, Randomized, Parallel group Efficacy and Safety Study for the Prevention of Venous Thromboembolism in Hospitalized Acutely Ill Medical Patients Comparing Rivaroxaban with Enoxaparin (MAGELLAN) trial evaluated 35-day therapy with rivaroxaban 10 mg daily versus standard 10-day therapy with enoxaparin [22]. While the rate of VTE was the same in both groups, major bleeding was increased in the extended duration rivaroxaban group. The Apixaban Dosing to Optimize Protection from Thrombosis (ADOPT) trial compared the novel oral anti-coagulant apixaban 5 mg daily with enoxaparin for extended duration thromboprophylaxis [25]. Thirty-day thromboprophylaxis with apixaban did not significantly decrease VTE compared with enoxaparin but did increase the frequency of major bleeding. The LIFENOX trial evaluated the effect of enoxaparin and compression stockings versus compression stockings alone on 30-day mortality in acutely ill medical patients [36]. Enoxaparin was not associated with a decrease in mortality after 30 days. The Discharge Alert Trial was a randomized controlled trial to test whether a hospital staff member's thromboprophylaxis alert to an Attending Physician prior to discharge would increase the rate of extended out-of-hospital prophylaxis and, in turn, reduce the incidence of symptomatic VTE at 90 days [37]. Physician alerts did not significantly decrease symptomatic VTE rates at 90 days. In aggregate, these five trials demonstrated no net clinical benefit with extended duration thromboprophylaxis in discharged medical patients. A currently-enrolling trial will evaluate the superiority of extended-duration anticoagulation with a factor Xa inhibitor betrixaban (for up to 35 days in hospital and post-discharge) compared with injectable enoxaparin (for 10 days) for VTE prevention in acute medically ill patients (ClinicalTrials.gov Identifier: NCT01583218). Another currently-enrolling trial will assess the efficacy and safety of a 45-day course of rivaroxaban 10 or 7.5 mg orally once daily versus placebo for prevention of symptomatic VTE and VTE-related death in high-risk medically ill patients after hospital discharge (ClinicalTrials.gov Identifier: NCT02111564).

Orthopedic Patients

VTE risk among orthopedic surgery patients remains significantly elevated even after discharge from the hospital. Extended out-of-hospital prophylaxis with warfarin or LMWH has been established as safe and effective in the prevention of VTE among orthopedic surgery patients [31, 32, 38]. Fondaparinux (2.5 mg subcutaneously once daily) has been shown to safely reduce the risk of VTE in patients undergoing hip replacement, major knee surgery, and hip fracture repair [39–42]. The American College of Chest Physicians (ACCP) Evidence-Based Clinical Practice Guidelines for Prevention of VTE in Orthopedic Surgery Patients also condones the use of aspirin for VTE prophylaxis in patients undergoing major orthopedic surgery [2].

Novel oral anticoagulants, including dabigatran [21], rivaroxaban [23, 24], apixiban [26, 27], and edoxaban [28] have been shown to be safe and effective for VTE prevention after orthopedic surgery. However, only rivaroxaban (10 mg orally daily) is currently approved by the U.S. Food and Drug Administration (FDA) for VTE prevention following knee or hip arthroplasty.

In an open-label, parallel-group study, investigators randomly assigned 300 patients undergoing elective unilateral total knee arthroplasty to receive either 200 or 300 mg daily of an antisense oligonucleotide that specifically reduces factor XI levels (FXI-ASO) or enoxaparin 40 mg daily [29]. The primary efficacy outcome of symptomatic VTE or DVT assessed by mandatory bilateral venography occurred in 27 % of patients who received the 200 mg dose of FXI-ASO and in 4 % of those who received the 300 mg dose, compared with 30 % of those who received enoxaparin. The 200 mg regimen was non-inferior, while the 300 mg regimen was superior compared with enoxaparin ($p < 0.001$). The frequency of bleeding was similar in both the FXI-ASO groups (3 and 3 %) but lower than that of the enoxaparin group (8 %).

Abdominal or Pelvic Surgery for Malignancy

Patients who have undergone abdominal or pelvic surgery for malignancy have a significantly elevated risk of postoperative VTE that extends past hospital discharge. In the Enoxaparin and Cancer (ENOXACAN) II study, extended-duration prophylaxis with enoxaparin significantly reduced the risk of VTE in patients undergoing laparotomy for abdominal or pelvic cancer [30].

Medical Oncology Patients

VTE is a common complication of cancer and chemotherapy [43, 44]. The frequency of symptomatic VTE in patients with malignancy during hospitalization ranges from 2 to 4 % and remains high, especially in the month following cancer diagnosis [43–45]. Validated risk stratification tools are available to identify cancer patients at particularly high risk for VTE (Table 13.1) [46].

Table 13.1 A generally accepted risk assessment tool for venous thromboembolism (VTE) in cancer patients

Patient characteristic	Points
Site of cancer	
Very high risk (stomach, pancreas)	2
High risk (lung, lymphoma, gynecologic, bladder, testicular)	1
Prechemotherapy platelet count ≥350,000/μL	1
Hemoglobin <10 g/dL or use of erythropoietic stimulating agents	1
Prechemotherapy leukocyte count >11,000/μL	1
Body mass index ≥35 kg/m²	1
"High risk" ≥3 points	

A randomized controlled trial of 1166 ambulatory patients receiving chemotherapy for metastatic or locally advanced solid cancer assessed the clinical benefit of the LMWH nadroparin for thromboprophylaxis [47]. Patients were randomly assigned to receive subcutaneous injections of nadroparin (3800 IU anti-Xa once a day) or placebo, in a 2:1 ratio. Seven hundred and sixty nine patients in the nadroparin group and 381 patients in the placebo group were included in the primary efficacy and safety analyses. Two percent of patients treated with nadroparin and 3.9 % of patients treated with placebo had a symptomatic venous or arterial thromboembolic event (single-sided p=0.02). There was no significant difference in major bleeding between the two groups.

An Overview of Prophylactic Regimens

The approach to VTE prevention among hospitalized and postoperative patients must consider the patient population and individual risk while integrating the use of mechanical and pharmacological modalities when indicated (Table 13.2).

Answer Key

1. **Correct answer**, (**c**) With the exception of prothrombin complex concentrate, which is used to reverse the anticoagulant effect of warfarin and the direct factor Xa inhibitors, all of the other interventions have reduced the frequency of VTE in randomized controlled trials of hospitalized patients.
2. **Correct answer**, (**b**) The American College of Physicians (ACP) Clinical Practice Guideline highlights assessment of risk for VTE and bleeding in all Medical Service patients prior to initiation of VTE prophylaxis as the most critical initial step in VTE prevention.

Table 13.2 Regimens for venous thromboembolism (VTE) prevention

Condition	Prophylaxis
General surgery	Unfractionated heparin 5000 units subcutaneously 2 or 3 times a day *or* Enoxaparin 40 mg subcutaneously daily *or* Dalteparin 2500 or 5000 units subcutaneously daily
Orthopedic surgery	Warfarin (target INR 2.0–3.0) *or* Enoxaparin 30 mg subcutaneously 2 times a day *or* Enoxaparin 40 mg subcutaneously daily *or* Dalteparin 2500 or 5000 units subcutaneously daily *or* Fondaparinux 2.5 mg subcutaneously daily *or* Rivaroxaban 10 mg orally daily *or* Aspirin 81–325 mg orally daily (often combined with mechanical prophylaxis)
Neurosurgery	Unfractionated heparin 5000 units subcutaneously 2 times a day *or* Enoxaparin 40 mg subcutaneously daily *and* Graduated compression stockings/intermittent pneumatic compression
Oncologic surgery	Enoxaparin 40 mg subcutaneously daily *or* Dalteparin 2500 or 5000 units subcutaneously daily
Thoracic surgery	Unfractionated heparin 5000 units subcutaneously 2–3 times a day *and* Graduated compression stockings/intermittent pneumatic compression
Medical patients	Unfractionated heparin 5000 units subcutaneously 2 or 3 times a day *or* Enoxaparin 40 mg subcutaneously daily *or* Dalteparin 2500 or 5000 units subcutaneously daily *or* Fondaparinux 2.5 mg subcutaneously daily (in patients with a heparin allergy such as heparin-induced thrombocytopenia) *or* Graduated compression stockings/intermittent pneumatic compression for patients with contraindications to anticoagulation Consider combination pharmacologic and mechanical prophylaxis for very-high-risk patients Consider surveillance lower extremity ultrasonography for intensive care unit patients

INR international normalized ratio

References

1. The surgeon general's call to action to prevent deep vein thrombosis and pulmonary embolism. U.S. Department of Health and Human Services. 2008. Available at: www.ncbi.nlm.nih.gov/books/NBK44178/. Accessed 21 Sept 2014.
2. Falck-Ytter Y, Francis CW, Johanson NA, et al. Prevention of VTE in orthopedic surgery patients: antithrombotic therapy and prevention of thrombosis, 9th ed: American College of Chest Physicians Evidence-Based Clinical Practice Guidelines. Chest. 2012;141:e278S–325.
3. Gould MK, Garcia DA, Wren SM, et al. Prevention of VTE in nonorthopedic surgical patients: antithrombotic therapy and prevention of thrombosis, 9th ed: American College of Chest Physicians Evidence-Based Clinical Practice Guidelines. Chest. 2012;141:e227S–77.
4. Kahn SR, Lim W, Dunn AS, et al. Prevention of VTE in nonsurgical patients: antithrombotic therapy and prevention of thrombosis, 9th ed: American College of Chest Physicians Evidence-Based Clinical Practice Guidelines. Chest. 2012;141:e195S–226.
5. Amin A, Stemkowski S, Lin J, Yang G. Thromboprophylaxis rates in US medical centers: success or failure? J Thromb Haemost. 2007;5:1610–6.

6. Kahn SR, Panju A, Geerts W, et al. Multicenter evaluation of the use of venous thromboembolism prophylaxis in acutely ill medical patients in Canada. Thromb Res. 2007;119:145–55.
7. Cohen AT, Tapson VF, Bergmann JF, et al. Venous thromboembolism risk and prophylaxis in the acute hospital care setting (ENDORSE study): a multinational cross-sectional study. Lancet. 2008;371:387–94.
8. Tapson VF, Decousus H, Pini M, et al. Venous thromboembolism prophylaxis in acutely ill hospitalized medical patients: findings from the International Medical Prevention Registry on Venous Thromboembolism. Chest. 2007;132:936–45.
9. Fiumara K, Piovella C, Hurwitz S, et al. Multi-screen electronic alerts to augment venous thromboembolism prophylaxis. Thromb Haemost. 2010;103:312–7.
10. Kucher N, Koo S, Quiroz R, et al. Electronic alerts to prevent venous thromboembolism among hospitalized patients. N Engl J Med. 2005;352:969–77.
11. Piazza G, Goldhaber SZ. Computerized decision support for the cardiovascular clinician: applications for venous thromboembolism prevention and beyond. Circulation. 2009;120:1133–7.
12. Piazza G, Goldhaber SZ. Physician alerts to prevent venous thromboembolism. J Thromb Thrombolysis. 2010;30:1–6.
13. Piazza G, Rosenbaum EJ, Pendergast W, et al. Physician alerts to prevent symptomatic venous thromboembolism in hospitalized patients. Circulation. 2009;119:2196–201.
14. Urbankova J, Quiroz R, Kucher N, Goldhaber SZ. Intermittent pneumatic compression and deep vein thrombosis prevention. A meta-analysis in postoperative patients. Thromb Haemost. 2005;94:1181–5.
15. Dennis M, Sandercock PA, Reid J, et al. Effectiveness of thigh-length graduated compression stockings to reduce the risk of deep vein thrombosis after stroke (CLOTS trial 1): a multicentre, randomised controlled trial. Lancet. 2009;373:1958–65.
16. CLOTS (Clots in Legs Or sTockings after Stroke) Trial Collaboration. Thigh-length versus below-knee stockings for deep venous thrombosis prophylaxis after stroke: a randomized trial. Ann Intern Med. 2010;153:553–62.
17. Dennis M, Sandercock P, Reid J, Graham C, Forbes J, Murray G. Effectiveness of intermittent pneumatic compression in reduction of risk of deep vein thrombosis in patients who have had a stroke (CLOTS 3): a multicentre randomised controlled trial. Lancet. 2013;382:516–24.
18. Qaseem A, Chou R, Humphrey LL, Starkey M, Shekelle P. Venous thromboembolism prophylaxis in hospitalized patients: a clinical practice guideline from the american college of physicians. Ann Intern Med. 2011;155:625–32.
19. Prevention of pulmonary embolism and deep vein thrombosis with low dose aspirin: Pulmonary Embolism Prevention (PEP) trial. Lancet. 2000;355:1295–302.
20. Cardiovascular Disease Educational and Research Trust; Cyprus Cardiovascular Disease Educational and Research Trust; European Venous Forum; International Surgical Thrombosis Forum; International Union of Angiology; Union Internationale de Phlébologie. Prevention and treatment of venous thromboembolism. International Consensus Statement (guidelines according to scientific evidence). Int Angiol. 2006;25:101–61.
21. Eriksson BI, Dahl OE, Rosencher N, et al. Dabigatran etexilate versus enoxaparin for prevention of venous thromboembolism after total hip replacement: a randomised, double-blind, non-inferiority trial. Lancet. 2007;370:949–56.
22. Cohen AT, Spiro TE, Buller HR, et al. Rivaroxaban for thromboprophylaxis in acutely ill medical patients. N Engl J Med. 2013;368:513–23.
23. Eriksson BI, Borris LC, Friedman RJ, et al. Rivaroxaban versus enoxaparin for thromboprophylaxis after hip arthroplasty. N Engl J Med. 2008;358:2765–75.
24. Kakkar AK, Brenner B, Dahl OE, et al. Extended duration rivaroxaban versus short-term enoxaparin for the prevention of venous thromboembolism after total hip arthroplasty: a double-blind, randomised controlled trial. Lancet. 2008;372:31–9.

25. Goldhaber SZ, Leizorovicz A, Kakkar AK, et al. Apixaban versus enoxaparin for thromboprophylaxis in medically ill patients. N Engl J Med. 2011;365:2167–77.
26. Lassen MR, Gallus A, Raskob GE, Pineo G, Chen D, Ramirez LM. Apixaban versus enoxaparin for thromboprophylaxis after hip replacement. N Engl J Med. 2010;363:2487–98.
27. Lassen MR, Raskob GE, Gallus A, Pineo G, Chen D, Hornick P. Apixaban versus enoxaparin for thromboprophylaxis after knee replacement (ADVANCE-2): a randomised double-blind trial. Lancet. 2010;375:807–15.
28. Raskob G, Cohen AT, Eriksson BI, et al. Oral direct factor Xa inhibition with edoxaban for thromboprophylaxis after elective total hip replacement. A randomised double-blind dose-response study. Thromb Haemost. 2010;104:642–9.
29. Buller HR, Bethune C, Bhanot S, et al. Factor XI antisense oligonucleotide for prevention of venous thrombosis. N Engl J Med. 2015;372:232–40.
30. Bergqvist D, Agnelli G, Cohen AT, et al. Duration of prophylaxis against venous thromboembolism with enoxaparin after surgery for cancer. N Engl J Med. 2002;346:975–80.
31. Eikelboom JW, Quinlan DJ, Douketis JD. Extended-duration prophylaxis against venous thromboembolism after total hip or knee replacement: a meta-analysis of the randomised trials. Lancet. 2001;358:9–15.
32. Hull RD, Pineo GF, Stein PD, et al. Extended out-of-hospital low-molecular-weight heparin prophylaxis against deep venous thrombosis in patients after elective hip arthroplasty: a systematic review. Ann Intern Med. 2001;135:858–69.
33. Hull RD, Schellong SM, Tapson VF, et al. Extended-duration venous thromboembolism prophylaxis in acutely ill medical patients with recently reduced mobility: a randomized trial. Ann Intern Med. 2010;153:8–18.
34. Dentali F, Douketis JD, Gianni M, Lim W, Crowther MA. Meta-analysis: anticoagulant prophylaxis to prevent symptomatic venous thromboembolism in hospitalized medical patients. Ann Intern Med. 2007;146:278–88.
35. Wein L, Wein S, Haas SJ, Shaw J, Krum H. Pharmacological venous thromboembolism prophylaxis in hospitalized medical patients: a meta-analysis of randomized controlled trials. Arch Intern Med. 2007;167:1476–86.
36. Kakkar AK, Cimminiello C, Goldhaber SZ, Parakh R, Wang C, Bergmann JF. Low-molecular-weight heparin and mortality in acutely ill medical patients. N Engl J Med. 2011; 365:2463–72.
37. Piazza G, Anderson FA, Ortel TL, et al. Randomized trial of physician alerts for thromboprophylaxis after discharge. Am J Med. 2013;126:435–42.
38. White RH, Gettner S, Newman JM, Trauner KB, Romano PS. Predictors of rehospitalization for symptomatic venous thromboembolism after total hip arthroplasty. N Engl J Med. 2000;343:1758–64.
39. Bauer KA, Eriksson BI, Lassen MR, Turpie AG. Fondaparinux compared with enoxaparin for the prevention of venous thromboembolism after elective major knee surgery. N Engl J Med. 2001;345:1305–10.
40. Eriksson BI, Bauer KA, Lassen MR, Turpie AG. Fondaparinux compared with enoxaparin for the prevention of venous thromboembolism after hip-fracture surgery. N Engl J Med. 2001;345:1298–304.
41. Turpie AG, Bauer KA, Eriksson BI, Lassen MR. Fondaparinux vs enoxaparin for the prevention of venous thromboembolism in major orthopedic surgery: a meta-analysis of 4 randomized double-blind studies. Arch Intern Med. 2002;162:1833–40.
42. Turpie AG, Gallus AS, Hoek JA. A synthetic pentasaccharide for the prevention of deep-vein thrombosis after total hip replacement. N Engl J Med. 2001;344:619–25.
43. Cronin-Fenton DP, Sondergaard F, Pedersen LA, et al. Hospitalisation for venous thromboembolism in cancer patients and the general population: a population-based cohort study in Denmark, 1997–2006. Br J Cancer. 2010;103:947–53.

44. Stein PD, Beemath A, Meyers FA, Skaf E, Sanchez J, Olson RE. Incidence of venous thromboembolism in patients hospitalized with cancer. Am J Med. 2006;119:60–8.
45. Khorana AA, Francis CW, Culakova E, Kuderer NM, Lyman GH. Frequency, risk factors, and trends for venous thromboembolism among hospitalized cancer patients. Cancer. 2007;110:2339–46.
46. Khorana AA, Connolly GC. Assessing risk of venous thromboembolism in the patient with cancer. J Clin Oncol. 2009;27:4839–47.
47. Agnelli G, Gussoni G, Bianchini C, et al. Nadroparin for the prevention of thromboembolic events in ambulatory patients with metastatic or locally advanced solid cancer receiving chemotherapy: a randomised, placebo-controlled, double-blind study. Lancet Oncol. 2009;10:943–9.

Appendix

Table 1 Characteristics of commonly used vasopressors and inotropes for hemodynamic support of patients with acute pulmonary embolism (PE)

Vasopressor/ inotrope	Mechanism of action	Dosing	Administration	Notes
Phenylephrine (Neosynephrine®)	Alpha-adrenergic agonist	Bolus: 100–500 mcg Infusion: 0–180 mcg/min	IV bolus and infusion	Pure vasoconstrictor; Helpful in PE patients with tachycardia
Norepinephrine (Levophed®)	Mixed alpha-/ beta-adrenergic agonist	Infusion: 0–30 mcg/min	IV infusion	May worsen tachycardia in PE patients
Ephedrine (Ephedrine)	Mixed alpha-/ beta-adrenergic agonist/ norepinephrine releasing agent	Bolus: 5–25 mg IVP, can be repeated every 5–10 min	IV bolus	Primarily used for post-anesthesia hypotension
Epinephrine (Adrenalin)	Mixed alpha-/ beta-adrenergic agonist	ACLS/bolus: 1 mg IVP, may be repeated every 3–5 min Infusion: 0–30 mcg/min;	IV bolus and infusion	May worsen tachycardia in PE patients
Vasopressin (Vasostrict®)	Vasopressin-receptor agonist	0.01–0.1 units/ min; ACLS dosing 40 units IV/IO push	IV infusion (bolus primarily for ACLS/ hemorrhagic shock)	Pure vasoconstrictor; may spare pulmonary vasculature; Helpful in PE patients with tachycardia

(continued)

© Springer International Publishing Switzerland 2015
G. Piazza et al., *Handbook for Venous Thromboembolism*,
DOI 10.1007/978-3-319-20843-5

Table 1 (continued)

Vasopressor/ inotrope	Mechanism of action	Dosing	Administration	Notes
Dopamine (Intropin®)	Mixed alpha-/ beta-adrenergic agonist	0–20 mcg/kg/ min	IV infusion	Degree of alpha and beta agonism dependent on dose of dopamine administered
Dobutamine (Dobutrex)	Beta-adrenergic agonist	Infusion: 0–20 mcg/kg/ min	IV infusion	May cause hypotension upon administration; May need to be paired with a vasoconstrictor
Milrinone (Primacor™)	Phosphodiesterase inhibitor/ ino-dilator	Infusion: 0.1–0.7 mcg/ kg/h	IV infusion	May cause hypotension upon administration; May need to be paired with a vasoconstrictor

IV intravenous, *ACLS* advanced cardiac life support, *IVP* intravenous push, *IO* intraosseous

Table 2 Characteristics of commonly used parenteral anticoagulants for venous thromboembolism (VTE) treatment

Anticoagulant	Mechanism of action	Standard dosing and dose adjustments	Administration	Elimination	Notes
Unfractionated heparin	Inhibition of factors II, V, VIII and X	Dosed by bolus and continuous infusion according to weight-based protocol; initial dosing for acute VTE: 80 units/kg ×1 followed by 18 units/kg/h titrated to a goal aPTT of 60–80 s	IV bolus and infusion	Primarily hepatic	Monitoring may be performed using aPTT or anti-Xa levels
Enoxaparin (Lovenox®)	LMWH; inhibition of factors II and X	1 mg/kg 2×/day or 1.5 mg/kg daily; CrCl<30 mL/min: 1 mg/kg daily	SC	40 % renal	Monitoring may be performed using anti-Xa levels (goal: 0.5–1.0 at 4–6 h after 2nd or 3rd dose); Monitoring is not routinely necessary; Not recommended in dialysis patients

Table 2 (continued)

Anticoagulant	Mechanism of action	Standard dosing and dose adjustments	Administration	Elimination	Notes
Dalteparin (Fragmin®)	LMWH; inhibition of factors II and X	200 IU/kg daily for 30 days followed by 150 IU/kg daily (maximum 18,000 IU); Renal dysfunction: adjust based on anti-Xa levels (goal 0.5–1.5 units/mL)	SC	Primarily renal	Monitoring may be performed using anti-Xa levels (goal: 0.5–1.0 at 4–6 h after 2nd or 3rd dose); Monitoring is not routinely necessary
Tinzaparin (Innohep®)	LMWH; inhibition of factors II and X	175 anti-Xa units/ kg daily;	SC	Primarily renal	Monitoring may be performed using anti-Xa levels; Monitoring is not routinely necessary; Use not recommended in patients with severe renal dysfunction
Fondaparinux (Arixtra®)	Direct factor Xa inhibitor	Weight-based dosing <50 kg: 5 mg daily 50–100 kg: 7.5 mg daily >100 kg: 10 mg daily	SC	80 % renal	Use not recommended in patients with renal dysfunction
Bivalirudin (Angiomax®)	Direct thrombin inhibitor	Dosed by continuous infusion according to weight-based protocol; 0.15–2 mg/kg/h and adjust to aPTT 1.5–2 times baseline	IV infusion	Primarily renal	Typically reserved for patients with suspected or confirmed HIT
Argatroban (Argatroban)	Direct thrombin inhibitor	Dosed by continuous infusion according to weight-based protocol; 1–2 mcg/ kg/min and adjust to aPTT 1.5–2 times baseline	IV infusion	Primarily hepatic	Typically reserved for patients with suspected or confirmed HIT

IV intravenous, *aPTT* activated partial thromboplastin time, *LMWH* low-molecular weight heparin, *SC* subcutaneous, *HIT* heparin-induced thrombocytopenia

Table 3 Characteristics of commonly used oral anticoagulants for venous thromboembolism (VTE) treatment

Anticoagulant	Mechanism of action	Dosing and dose adjustment	Elimination	Half-life	Notes
Warfarin (Coumadin®)	Inhibits vitamin K mediated gamma-carboxylation of factors II, VII, IX, X	Dosing based on INR; usual starting dose 5 mg daily	Primarily hepatic metabolism	30–40 h	Requires overlap ("bridging") with a parenteral anticoagulant for at least 5 days and until the INR is within target for two consecutive days
Dabigatran (Pradaxa™)	Direct thrombin inhibitor	150 mg PO 2×/day; CrCl 15–30 mL/min: 75 mg PO 2×/day	80 % renal	12–14 h	Requires 5–10 days of parenteral anticoagulation before switching to oral dabigatran
Rivaroxaban (Xarelto™)	Direct factor Xa inhibitor	15 mg PO 2×/day ×3 weeks, then 20 mg PO daily; CrCl <30 mL/min: use not recommended	35 % renal	6–9 h	Total oral monotherapy without need for parenteral anticoagulation lead-in
Apixaban (Eliquis™)	Direct factor Xa inhibitor	10 mg PO BID ×1 week, then 5 mg PO 2×/day; dose reduction-2.5 mg 2×/day if 2 or more of the following criteria are present: age >80, weight <60 kg, SCr >1.5; 2.5 mg 2×/day also available for extended duration anticoagulation to prevent recurrent VTE	30 % renal	8–12 h	Total oral monotherapy without need for parenteral anticoagulation lead-in
Edoxaban (Savaysa™)	Direct factor Xa inhibitor	60 mg PO daily; CrCl 15–50 mL/min: 30 mg PO daily	70 % renal	10–14 h	Caution in patients with CrCl >90; may increase risk of VTE due to increased drug clearance; Requires 5–10 days of parenteral anticoagulation before switching to oral edoxaban

INR international normalized ratio, *CrCl* creatinine clearance

Index

© Springer International Publishing Switzerland 2015
G. Piazza et al., *Handbook for Venous Thromboembolism*,
DOI 10.1007/978-3-319-20843-5

Printed by Printforce, the Netherlands